T0290877

Praise for
Unfolding Health Assessment Case Studies for the Student Nurse
Second Edition

"This is an extraordinary and contemporary learning resource for all nursing students and faculty. This book is logically organized and enhances the student learning experience by explaining and describing concepts that guide students in the application and retention of nursing knowledge, assessing various health conditions across the life span. The illustrations teach students the importance of detailed interviewing, data collection, and how to think through simple to complex nursing assessments when caring for diverse populations."

–Jeffery Ramirez, PhD, PMHNP-BC, CNE, FNAP, FAANP, FAAN
Director of Graduate Nursing Programs and Professor
Gonzaga University, School of Health Sciences

"This remarkable book prepares the nursing student for the rigors of clinical practice by integrating anatomy, physiology, health assessment, clinical presentation, and laboratory data in a compact, clean, yet comprehensive way. The ease of reading the 16 chapters cannot be overemphasized. This notable book will amplify essential 'knowing' for the newest to enter our profession. Quite simply, this little gem delivers!"

–Linda Honan, PhD, CNS-BC, FAAN, ANEF
Professor Emerita, Yale University School of Nursing

Praise for the first edition of
Unfolding Health Assessment Case Studies for the Student Nurse

"This book is a must-have resource for health assessment educators and their students. Utilizing this text, students will be challenged to apply health assessment concepts and develop important critical-thinking skills. The use of unfolding case studies with NCLEX-style practice questions is extremely useful and can be effective both inside and outside the classroom. This will be a well-loved and dog-eared text on many a bookshelf for years to come."

–Maryanne Davidson, DNSc, APRN, CPNP
Dean, St. Vincent's College, Sacred Heart University

UNFOLDING
HEALTH ASSESSMENT
CASE STUDIES
FOR THE STUDENT NURSE

SECOND EDITION

KRISTI MAYNARD, EdD, APRN, FNP-BC, CNE

ANDREA ADIMANDO, DNP, MSN, MS, APRN, PMHNP-BC, BCIM

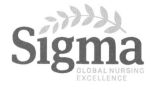

Sigma
GLOBAL NURSING
EXCELLENCE

Sigma Theta Tau International Honor Society of Nursing (Sigma) is a nonprofit organization whose mission is developing nurse leaders anywhere to improve healthcare everywhere. Founded in 1922, Sigma has more than 135,000 active members in over 100 countries and territories. Members include practicing nurses, instructors, researchers, policymakers, entrepreneurs, and others. Sigma's more than 540 chapters are located at more than 700 institutions of higher education throughout Armenia, Australia, Botswana, Brazil, Canada, Chile, Colombia, Croatia, England, Eswatini, Finland, Ghana, Hong Kong, Ireland, Israel, Italy, Jamaica, Japan, Jordan, Kenya, Lebanon, Malawi, Mexico, the Netherlands, Nigeria, Pakistan, Philippines, Portugal, Puerto Rico, Scotland, Singapore, South Africa, South Korea, Sweden, Taiwan, Tanzania, Thailand, the United States, and Wales. Learn more at www.sigmanursing.org.

Sigma Theta Tau International
550 West North Street
Indianapolis, IN, USA 46202

To request a review copy for course adoption, order additional books, buy in bulk, or purchase for corporate use, contact Sigma Marketplace at 888.654.4968 (US/Canada toll-free), +1.317.687.2256 (International), or solutions@sigmamarketplace.org.

To request author information, or for speaker or other media requests, contact Sigma Marketing at 888.634.7575 (US/Canada toll-free) or +1.317.634.8171 (International).

ISBN: 9781646481309
EPUB ISBN: 9781646481316
PDF ISBN: 9781646481330

Library of Congress Control Number: 2024002769

Publisher: Dustin Sullivan
Acquisitions Editor: Emily Hatch
Development Editor: Jillmarie Leeper Sycamore
Cover Designer: Rebecca Batchelor
Interior Design/Page Layout: Bumpy Design
Indexer: Larry D. Sweazy
Managing Editor: Carla Hall
Publications Specialist: Todd Lothery
Project Editor: Todd Lothery
Copy Editor: Todd Lothery
Proofreaders: Jane Palmer, Julie Siegel

About the Authors

Kristi Maynard, EdD, APRN, FNP-BC, CNE, is an American Nurses Credentialing Center (ANCC) board-certified advanced practice registered nurse in the specialty area of family practice (FNP). She also achieved certification through the National League for Nursing as a certified nurse educator (CNE). She received her BSN from Mount Saint Mary College in Newburgh, New York, and her MSN from Fairfield University in Fairfield, Connecticut.

She began her career in nursing more than 15 years ago as a medical intensive care nurse. After graduating with her MSN, she entered full-time practice as an FNP in the primary care environment. She remains active in clinical practice in her independently owned and operated primary care practice. Currently, she is an Associate Professor of Nursing at Southern Connecticut State University and the lead family nurse practitioner faculty for their FNP program. She teaches in both the graduate and undergraduate nursing programs with a course load focused on health assessment, health assessment lab, pathophysiology, and pharmacology. In addition to her authorship, she contracts as an editorial consultant for nursing and nurse practitioner test bank content.

Andrea Adimando, DNP, MSN, MS, APRN, PMHNP-BC, BCIM, is an Associate Professor of Nursing and Director of the MSN program at Southern Connecticut State University. She is an ANCC board-certified psychiatric-mental health nurse practitioner (PMHNP-BC) and a former pediatric medical-surgical nurse. She earned a bachelor's degree in behavioral neuroscience from Lehigh University in 2003 and a master of science in nursing from Yale School of Nursing in 2006. She later earned a master of science in human nutrition from the University of Bridgeport in 2012 and a DNP from Chatham University in 2014.

In addition to her clinical practice, Adimando has published several peer-reviewed articles and presented at local and national conferences on her research interests. These include complementary and alternative therapies, multimodal educational strategies for nursing students, and compassion fatigue in nurses. She has also previously served as the Vice Chairperson on the ANCC's content expert panel for the PMHNP board certification exam, as well as a member of the panel for eight years. Recently, she received the ANCC's prestigious Certified Nurse Award for her contributions as a PMHNP in Connecticut.

Adimando has over 15 years of pediatric and psychiatric nursing experience and continues to practice as a PMHNP in various levels of care across Connecticut. Within her previous positions in emergency psychiatry, inpatient and outpatient psychiatry, her private practice, and pediatric medical-surgical settings, she focused on the integration and interdependence of physical and mental health. The health assessment skills she acquired through this expansive background allow her to apply real-life clinical scenarios and relevant expertise to her teaching of health assessment to BSN and MSN students.

Contributing Authors

Ashley Dobuzinsky, DNP, MSN, RN, CNEcl, is a registered nurse in the specialty of emergency nursing. She received her associate of science in nursing in 2005 from St. Vincent's College in Bridgeport, Connecticut, and a bachelor of science in nursing in 2010 from Southern Connecticut State University in New Haven. She earned a master of science in nursing education from the University of Hartford and a DNP from Capella University in Minneapolis, Minnesota. She is also certified by the National League for Nursing as an academic clinical nurse educator (CNEcl).

Dobuzinsky has over 18 years of nursing experience and began her career as a critical care nurse, working in a mixed medical-surgical and cardiothoracic intensive care unit. She has also served as a designated rapid response team nurse. As a nurse educator, she has held roles as a service line educator for the Department of Cardiology at St. Vincent's Medical Center in Bridgeport and an adjunct clinical instructor for St. Vincent's College at Sacred Heart University. She currently serves as a bedside nurse in the emergency department at Griffin Hospital in Derby, Connecticut.

Louis E. D'Onofrio Jr., DNP, MSN, FNP-C, PCCN, is the founder of Best Health Primary Care, a medical practice located in Stratford, Connecticut, founded in 2016. Before devoting his work to providing high-quality primary care services, D'Onofrio was a medical intensive care unit nurse and charge nurse at Yale-New Haven Hospital. He completed his bachelor's degree at the Catholic University of America in Washington, DC, a master's degree at Fairfield University, and a doctorate at the University of Arkansas. D'Onofrio also holds the position of Clinical Care Director at the Westport Weston Health District in Westport, Connecticut.

Carrie D. Michalski, JD, MSN, RN, began her nursing career in New York City as a BSN graduate in labor and delivery, quickly gaining skills in all facets of maternal, child, and women's health. As she started to focus on the medico-legal aspects of OB/GYN care, she attained a JD, thereafter specializing in medical malpractice litigation defense. Additional opportunities presented while consulting at culturally diverse community health centers, which offered a range of roles from administrative to education and patient care. Her legal, business, and healthcare lens offers a unique nursing perspective. Since 2002, Michalski has been teaching at the BSN level across the nursing curriculum in lecture, labs, simulation, and clinical. Her master of nursing education degree informs her research interests in the scholarship of teaching and learning. She strives to understand and improve the student experience and assists in students' transition to practice.

Vanessa Pomarico, EdD, APRN, FNP-BC, FAANP, is senior faculty for Fitzgerald Health Education Associates. She is the Lead Clinician for Diversity and Inclusion at Northeast Medical Group, with a special interest in LGBTQIA+ healthcare. An author, lecturer, educator, and volunteer, Pomarico is the former Director and Lead Faculty of the FNP track in the Department of Nursing at Southern Connecticut State University. She is courtesy faculty and a guest lecturer for several nurse practitioner, physician assistant, and medical schools in Connecticut. She is the recipient of numerous awards including the American Association of Nurse Practitioners Nurse Practitioner Excellence Award, the Nightingale Award for Excellence in Nursing, and the YNHH APC Clinical Excellence Award. She has served as the Co-chair of Health Policy and is a Past President of the Connecticut Advanced Practice Registered Nurse Society and presents at local and national conferences.

Dilice Robertson, DNP, MSN, APRN, PMHCNS-BC, PMHNP-BC, is a Clinical Associate Professor at NYU Meyers College of Nursing and previous faculty member at Fairfield University and Yale University School of Nursing. She was the inaugural faculty chair delegate of the Yale School of Nursing IDEAS (Inclusion, Diversity, Equity, Action, Solutions) council, the organization that champions diversity, equity, and inclusion within the school.

Robertson has received many awards, including the Annie Goodrich Award for Excellence in Teaching, and is the founder of a group psychiatric-mental health practice in Connecticut. She sits on two nonprofit boards in Connecticut, for one of which she is board chair. She works with elementary schools implementing programs to improve emotional and behavioral regulation in youth through social-emotional and mindfulness curricula to reduce the potential for development of mental health disorders.

Antoinette Towle, EdD, MSN, APRN, SNP-BC, PNP-BC, is an Associate Professor in the Nursing Department at Southern Connecticut State University in New Haven, Connecticut. She is an American Nurses Credentialing Center board-certified advanced practice registered nurse in the specialty areas of pediatric and school health. Towle has worked as a professional nurse for over 30 years in a variety of capacities (administrator, nursing home owner, manager, director, caseworker, APRN, RN, and educator) and within a wide variety of healthcare settings (acute and chronic care hospitals; schools; residential settings for children, adolescents, and the elderly; VA hospitals; insurance companies; federal and privately funded medical offices; and community healthcare agencies). She presently teaches full time both graduate and undergraduate nursing students with focus on nursing leadership; understanding, respecting, and appreciating cultural diversity; health promotion; and integration of these key components into clinical practice. She was the first to create and continues to lead a nursing study abroad service in Jamaica, China, Nicaragua, Peru, and Armenia.

Tammy Wen-Chun Lo, MSN, APRN, ACNP-BC, earned a bachelor's degree in neurobiology, physiology, and behavior from the University of California, Davis; she later transitioned to nursing via the Graduate Entry Pre-specialty in Nursing Program at the Yale School of Nursing. She earned her master of nursing at Yale with a focus on adult acute care. After working in neurosurgery for several years, she joined Nuvance Health, formerly Western Connecticut Health Network, as part of a pancreatic cancer screening clinical trial involving hereditary high-risk individuals as well as individuals with new-onset diabetes. Her article "Screening for Pancreatic Cancer in Individuals With New-Onset Diabetes Mellitus" won the inaugural Marilyn Edmunds Journal for Nurse Practitioners Writing Award in 2019.

Additional Book Resources

To download a sample chapter and other free book resources, visit the Sigma Repository at https://sigma.nursingrepository.org/handle/10755/23577 or scan the QR code.

Facilitator Guide Available

A facilitator guide is available from Sigma Marketplace and as a print product from most online book retailers. Simply search for this book title with the added keywords of "facilitator guide" to purchase it. You can also email our Marketplace team for bulk orders at solutions@sigmamarketplace.org.

Special Note to Readers

Here at Sigma, we realize that language is constantly evolving. The meaning of a word often changes over time, some words become obsolete, and some terms that were once acceptable may become controversial or even offensive, depending on the context or circumstances. We have made every effort to make language choices that are inclusive and not offensive. Should you identify words in this book that you believe negatively impact a group or groups of people, please reach out to us at Publications@SigmaNursing.org.

Table of Contents

Introduction

Welcome, student nurse readers and educators alike, to what we hope will be an enlightening, informative, and fun addition to your nursing school textbook collection. We are so thankful for the positive response to the first edition of this book and are thrilled to have the opportunity to release a second edition of this text! We recognize that the climate of healthcare and nursing education is changing. In schools of nursing across the country, there is an increased focus on developing clinical judgment to increase the quality of patient care for graduate nurses entering practice. The stakes have never been higher as nursing shortages rage on in the wake of COVID-19. We hope this book can contribute as a low-fidelity tool to build student knowledge and confidence in the understanding of health assessment.

The new edition includes three new chapters to further assist in the pursuit of nursing knowledge. Chapter 4 helps students tackle the basics of the patient interview and introduces emerging technologies. Chapter 5 focuses on the basics of gathering and interpreting vital signs across the life span, and Chapter 6 introduces the student to mental status assessment. Another exciting feature of this edition is the expanded practice test. The revised test includes a collection of NextGen-style questions, in addition to those in the chapters, to help better prepare students for coursework, boards, and, of course, practice! To help get started, Chapter 3 now includes samples and descriptions of NextGen-style questions in addition to traditional NCLEX question formats.

This book can be used by early-career nursing students who have just begun to cover its concepts as well as by prelicensure exam students who may benefit from reiteration and reinforcement of concepts learned early on in nursing school—and from practicing applying these concepts to more complex scenarios.

We hope that our readers will utilize our book to attain the following knowledge and/or skills:

- Increased comfort level and confidence in analyzing patient scenarios in regard to basic health assessment

- A more in-depth knowledge of basic health assessment concepts
- Ample chances to practice applying concepts learned in your health assessment course to solidify the information you have learned
- Increased confidence in answering NCLEX and NextGen-style questions
- Increased knowledge, skill levels, and confidence in assessing and managing patients with diverse healthcare needs

The chapters of the book do not have to be completed in any particular order, as they are each individualized to certain subject matter categories. We recommend you use these unfolding case studies as a means of evaluating the ability to think critically and apply the concepts learned in health assessment class to realistic patient scenarios. The book can be used as a study tool during health assessment class, a health assessment refresher during other classes, and/or an NCLEX study tool at the end of the nursing school journey.

Introduction to the Unfolding Case Study

Kristi Maynard, EdD, APRN, FNP-BC, CNE

Welcome to *Unfolding Health Assessment Case Studies for the Student Nurse,* 2nd Edition! Purchasing this book was your first step in mastering the concepts of nursing health assessment. It will introduce general principles of assessment, highlight key facts and information, and provide you with guidance on approaching NCLEX-style questions.

Chapter 1 covers some basic information that will help you maximize the use of this book as part of your learning process.

Health Assessment Skills: Putting It Together

As a nursing student, health assessment can seem overwhelming. There is so much to know and even more to *understand*. You may be wondering what the difference is. Well, *learning* something means you can recall it, but *understanding* something means you can not only recall information but also apply it. You can think critically about advanced concepts and apply what you know to make informed decisions for your patient's care. This will help you not only be a more successful student nurse but also progress to a more informed professional nurse.

Health assessment is one of the first courses where you are putting it all together. You are taking the information you have learned in all your foundational courses and beginning the process of critical analysis, which is imperative for your development as a professional nurse. For

 What is the NCLEX?

The National Council Licensure Examination (NCLEX) is the nationwide licensure examination used in the United States. The NCLEX is developed and administered by the National Council of State Boards of Nursing. Once you graduate from your nursing program, you are required to meet the minimum passing requirements of the NCLEX before you can apply for state licensure. The exam ensures that you are competent to enter professional practice as an entry-level nurse.

the first time, you will consider why something is happening. For example, *intermittent claudication* is defined as pain in the legs while walking. As discussed, it is not enough to merely know the definition; you must understand why the symptom occurs and reflect on what it reveals about your patient's health condition.

As an experienced nurse, I can logically deduce that if my patient subjectively reports symptoms consistent with intermittent claudication, the patient is probably experiencing oxygen starvation in the muscles of the legs when walking. This is likely because the muscles are not receiving adequate blood flow, which is generally caused by plaque development in the major arterial vessels of the legs (because I know arteries carry oxygenated blood). Now that I have identified a potential cause, I can let that lead the rest of my physical assessment. I should consider checking pulses, examining skin quality for ulcerations and temperature, or auscultating for femoral bruits.

Health assessment is like developing a superpower. Based on the subjective and objective information you gather from your patient, you are able to predict patient needs, anticipate impending disaster, and deduce precise elements of your patient's health. As a student nurse, understanding the basics and being able to apply the information you gather to contribute to the big picture will help you during your academic career.

With a solid foundation in critical reasoning and application, you can recall your health assessment roots to think through more complex scenarios that will arise through your nursing education. If you fail to master this content, it is likely you will struggle to build your nursing knowledge. You must lay a solid foundation before you put up the walls. The comprehensive, head-to-toe health assessment is a rite of passage. The ability to perform a head-to-toe assessment in a calculated, meaningful way means you have arrived!

The Traditional Case Study

A *case study* is the presentation of a patient scenario meant to illustrate a particular concept or principle. Case studies may vary in length and complexity. Some may ask you to answer a set of questions at the end; others may provide you with the answers to pertinent questions for the sake of delivering specific content. The overarching goal of the case study is to engage the reader in the critical analysis of the patient scenario. Case studies are very popular in the field of nursing, but they are not unique to the nursing community. They are frequently used in the social sciences.

While there are some variations in exactly how they may appear, case studies are a widely accepted method incorporated into nursing education to engage the student in the process of active learning. *Active learning* is the process of learning in an engaged, interactive format that invokes critical thinking. Inversely, *passive learning* is when you are learning despite a lack of critical thinking or active engagement. An example of passive learning might be listening to a traditional lecture with accompanying PowerPoint. Evidence-based literature tells us that active learning is superior for long-term recall and application (Prince, 2004). Engaging in active learning strategies greatly increases the likelihood that you are not simply recalling information on cue but that you truly understand the information and can apply it to complex situations.

The Unfolding Case Study

Similar to a traditional case study, an *unfolding case study* presents the reader with a patient scenario. What is unique about the unfolding case study is the evolutionary nature of the scenario. This simulated scenario provides readers with more information about the patient or the patient's progress as they work through the case. This is beneficial because it allows for the case to begin with basic concepts and layer more complex concepts as the case builds. Using this method, readers must not only consider what has already happened but also anticipate potential changes in patient status.

This process of evaluation and reevaluation is more consistent with real-life patient care and aids in the development of clinical reasoning skills (Bowman, 2017). As a method of low-fidelity simulation, the unfolding case study has been recognized by the National League for Nursing as a robust and meaningful student learning experience (National League for Nursing, 2019).

Integrating unfolding case studies into your study routine means integrating simulation. Simulation has become a critical element of nursing education (Eyikara & Baykara, 2017). When you think of simulation, you probably imagine a simulation lab with high-tech mannequins and lots of fancy equipment—*high-fidelity simulation*.

What you probably don't realize is that you can engage in simulation activities from the comfort of your own home with no high-tech mannequins required! *Low-fidelity simulation* involves simulated patient scenarios with little or no technological component. Sound familiar?

Unfolding case studies are the perfect example of a low-fidelity simulation activity. Like high-fidelity simulation, these cases ask the reader to engage in critical reasoning and active learning, two methods known to increase a student's ability to comprehend and apply the content they are studying (Sofer, 2018). *Critical reasoning* involves the ability to actively and skillfully conceptualize, analyze, question, and evaluate a scenario and is imperative for both the NCLEX and professional nursing success.

The unfolding case study is a form of active learning. It requires repetitive evaluation and reevaluation of the patient scenario to determine health outcomes and nursing priorities. The unfolding case study is a method of low-fidelity simulation, which means it doesn't require any fancy, expensive equipment!

Active learning activities will better prepare you to apply elements of critical reasoning when presented with either a fictional or, more importantly, real-life scenario. To put it simply, you will be better prepared to think on your feet if you have prepared with active learning strategies. So, when those NCLEX questions are asking you to select the "most correct" response, you will be able to meaningfully analyze the stem and responses and make the correct choice because that is what you have been training yourself to do all along! If you have been relying on methods of recall to get you through nursing school, complex NCLEX questions that ask you to analyze and interpret a scenario may seem impossible.

The case studies in this text have been developed with the novice nursing student in mind. They are purposefully simplified to match your current level of application while still offering lessons in critical reasoning to enhance not only health assessment skills but your practical skills. Whenever you are engaged in active learning, you are building your practical and clinical reasoning skills.

Tips for Working With Unfolding Case Studies

Here are a few tips for getting the most out of the unfolding case studies presented in this book:

Read each case carefully.

Put the book down for a few seconds after reading a new section of the vignette (the case), and think about how what you just read will affect your patient. How does this influence your plan of care? What are your priorities for care? Have your priorities changed based on the information you just read?

Don't jump ahead to the practice questions.

Be thoughtful about the patient scenario and consider the details you have been presented. Health assessment is about taking in the subjective and objective information that you gather and formulating priorities and a plan based on evidence-based best practice for patient care. We will integrate evidence-based practices throughout the cases.

Read the questions carefully.

Underline key components of the question and then carefully read through the options. Think. It. Through. Simplify the question in your own words to make it more manageable (keeping scrap paper close by is helpful).

Read through the question rationale.

Take the time to read and understand why your selection was correct or incorrect. Make notes or comments on the page that help you identify and retain key pieces of information that may be helpful in your future studies. If you read a rationale and still find yourself uncertain about content or a concept, look it up! Use your textbook or an evidence-based search engine to get more information on what you are investigating.

Look through a new lens.

After you have completed the guidance questions, go back to the previous section of the vignette and read through it again. Now that you have acquired new knowledge, were there key elements in the patient description that might have led you to prioritize this patient differently?

Think ahead and take a moment to ask, "What if?"

Based on the current state and trajectory of your patient, what do you anticipate may happen to this patient in the future? How might that affect your nursing priorities or care?

Set yourself up for success!

Don't get discouraged or frustrated if you don't know the answer to a question. This is a tool for learning; it is not expected that you will answer every question perfectly. The questions are intended to provide practice with NCLEX-style questions while introducing relevant content.

Conclusion

Each chapter ends with a worksheet (see Sample Worksheet at the end of this chapter). The worksheet contains prompts to direct your thoughts and help you identify areas of strength and weakness. Use these worksheets to realistically evaluate your performance on the case. Self-evaluation is a valuable tool for personal growth.

In closing, have fun with this book. We hope it serves as the powerful study resource we intend it to be. As nursing professors who have been teaching undergraduate health assessment for many years, we appreciate the complexity of this material. We understand how much easier it is to understand and apply this content if it is presented in a way that gets you thinking, and we hope this text does just that!

SAMPLE WORKSHEET

Based on my initial assessment, I thought:

_____

_____

_____

Based on my revised/informed assessment, I now know:

_____

_____

_____

A nursing priority for this patient would be _____

because _____

After completing this chapter, something I have learned is:

_____

_____

_____

After completing this chapter, something I need more clarity on is:

_____

_____

_____

After completing this chapter, something else I want to learn is:

_____

_____

_____

REFERENCES

Bowman, K. (2017). Use of online unfolding case studies to foster critical thinking. *Journal of Nursing Education, 56*(11), 701–702. https://doi.org/10.3928/01484834-20171020-13

Eyikara, E., & Baykara, Z. G. (2017). The importance of simulation in nursing education. *World Journal on Educational Technology: Current Issues, 9*(1), 2–7.

National League for Nursing. (2019). *ACE.Z unfolding cases.* https://www.nln.org/education/ teaching-resources/professional-development-programsteaching-resourcesace-all/ace-z/ unfolding-cases-7798b55c-7836-6c70-9642-ff00005f0421

Prince, M. (2004). Does active learning work? A review of the research. *Journal of Engineering Education, 93*(3), 223–231.

Sofer, D. (2018). The value of simulation in nursing education. *American Journal of Nursing, 118*(4), 17–18. https://doi.org/10.1097/01.NAJ.0000532063.79102.19

CHAPTER 2

Introduction to the Nursing Process

Andrea Adimando, DNP, MSN, MS, APRN, PMHNP-BC, BCIM

The nursing process was developed in 1958 by Ida Jean Orlando, and it continues to be an essential component of nursing education and practice to this day. It is a five-step process (see Figure 2.1) that provides a framework for nurses to identify and treat actual or potential health problems in an individualized, patient-centered manner. The nursing process consists of five basic steps (Potter et al., 2017):

1. Assessment
2. Diagnosis
3. Planning (sometimes referred to as Outcomes and Planning)
4. Implementation
5. Evaluation

Understanding the nursing process is key to critical thinking and problem-solving in nursing practice. Each of these steps is described in detail in this chapter and will also be referenced in Chapter 3 in regard to preparing to answer NCLEX-style questions. However, for the purposes of this book, the primary focus is on the assessment phase of the nursing process.

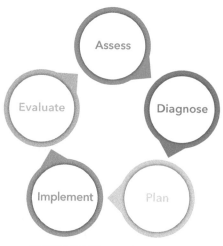

FIGURE 2.1 The nursing process.

Assessment

The first step, *assessment,* is a critical part of the nursing process that involves subjective and objective data collection. Subjective data can be collected via multiple means, including patient reports (verbal statements from patient or caregiver) and patient history (either by report or by chart review). Ways of measuring objective data include vital signs, intake and output, pain scales, and lab values. The purpose of the assessment phase is to collect all data that may be pertinent to formulating a nursing diagnosis and/or to assist in the provider's formulation of a medical diagnosis, as well as to prepare for implementation of care measures that are individualized to the patient you have assessed (Potter et al., 2017; Toney-Butler & Thayer, 2019).

Another reason that assessment is key to the nursing process is that this phase requires critical thinking skills to be employed right from the start of your patient care. As you continue to collect assessment data, you should already be thinking about how these data may play into your care plan for your particular patient and how you will continue to assess your patient (subjectively and objectively) throughout all steps of the nursing process. Not only does the assessment phase focus on the collection of data but also the validation and interpretation of that information to ensure it is accurate and complete (Potter et al., 2017).

As you make your way through this text, you will quickly notice that the assessment phase is its primary focus. It is essential to master assessment early on in your nursing student journey to ensure that you can comfortably and safely move on to diagnosing and planning care for your patients in an informed and patient-centered way.

Diagnosis

After you have completed the assessment phase—gathering data from subjective and objective sources, verifying and documenting the data, and beginning to analyze the data—you can move on to the diagnosis phase of the nursing process. The *diagnosis* phase involves critically thinking and analyzing your data to formulate a nursing clinical judgment. According to Potter et al. (2017), "A nursing diagnosis is a clinical judgment concerning a human response to health conditions/life processes, or vulnerability for that response by an individual, family, or community that a nurse is licensed and competent to treat" (p. 225). In this quote, "competent to treat" refers to nurses formulating diagnoses that are related to their scope of practice as nurses, that they are then able to manage via nursing interventions. This differs from a medical diagnosis in that a medical diagnosis (e.g., diabetes mellitus, Alzheimer's disease, etc.) is based on a set of symptoms that remains relatively consistent throughout treatment. A nursing diagnosis is generally more fluid, able to be "resolved" by the nurse with careful nursing planning and implementation (Chiffi & Zanotti, 2014).

In addition to standard nursing diagnoses, you may also create your own diagnoses based on your own knowledge that is correlated with the patient experience. When identifying and validating a nursing diagnosis, it is important to ensure that (Herdman et al., 2021):

- The majority of the defining characteristics and/or risk factors are present in the patient.
- The etiological factors for the diagnosis are evident in your patient.
- You have validated the diagnosis with the patient/family or with a nurse peer (when possible).

While it will take some time for you to become accustomed to formulating and documenting nursing diagnoses, you will quickly learn that having a solid collection of nursing diagnoses for a patient can significantly improve their treatment and outcomes. Only when nurses are cooperating as a team to address these patient needs from a nursing standpoint, as well as working collaboratively with other disciplines, can optimal patient care be achieved.

Creating a nursing diagnosis is often referred to as "diagnostic reasoning" in nursing education. In *diagnostic reasoning,* a clinical nursing judgment is formulated based on the information at hand (gathered during the assessment phase), with the goal of individualizing patient care planning based on this judgment. Diagnoses are formed by collecting and collating data; analyzing health strengths, vulnerabilities, and needs of the patient; and labeling these with related nursing diagnoses (Nurjannah et al., 2013).

Planning

Once nurses have transitioned their assessment findings into a set of nursing diagnoses, they can move on to the *planning* phase of the nursing process. In this phase, the nurse uses critical thinking skills to create a care plan that is individualized to the particular patient's needs and current health status. The plan is also tailored to a framework that is based on a particular outcome or set of outcomes that is the goal for that patient. For this reason, this phase is sometimes referred to as the "outcomes planning" phase.

Typically, patients in the acute care (hospital) setting have more than one problem that needs to be addressed. Patients can have multiple problems, as well as multiple medical and nursing diagnoses, many of which may have been present on admission and some of which may have developed over the course of a hospitalization (think hospital-acquired infections, bedsores, etc.). For this reason, it is important for nurses to prioritize these needs during the planning phase. By prioritizing patient health as well as spiritual and psychological needs, the nursing care team can improve the safety and effectiveness of their nursing care and ultimately improve outcomes for their patients.

Table 2.1 shows a series of nursing diagnoses for which the nurse has planned goals and expected outcomes for a patient who is postoperative.

TABLE 2.1 Nursing Diagnoses, Goals, and Expected Outcomes for the Postoperative Patient

Nursing Diagnoses	Goals	Outcomes Expected
Pain related to surgery	Mrs. Radiant will achieve pain relief by day of discharge.	Pt reports pain at a level of < 4 by day of discharge. Pt transfers from bed to chair with no increase in pain in 48 hours.
Knowledge deficit related to impending discharge	Mrs. Radiant will express understanding of post-operative risks. Mrs. Radiant will verbalize self-care needs.	Pt verbalizes home activity restrictions by day of discharge. Pt verbalizes knowledge and demonstrates skill of cleaning incision by day of discharge. Pt describes risks for infection within one day of surgery.
Risk for infection	Mrs. Radiant will remain infection-free while in the hospital.	Patient remains afebrile while in the hospital. Patient's incision shows no signs of infection. Pt incisional area shows signs of healing and closure by day of discharge.

(Adapted from Potter et al., 2017)

As you can see from Table 2.1, all goals are directly related to the nursing diagnoses and are measurable and attainable. If goals are not attainable, the care plan will not be successful, and the objectives will not be met. This often requires critical thinking and careful reassessment in order to achieve. The expected outcomes also match the diagnoses and the goals, and they should be reasonable and measurable as well.

Implementation

Implementation refers to the phase where the nurse begins to employ treatment strategies and interventions to achieve the goals and identified outcomes in the patient care plan. These interventions may be nurse-driven, or they may be more collaborative interventions that involve the care team or the therapeutic acute care or milieu environment(s) (Potter et al., 2017).

Prior to implementing an intervention, the nurse must know the reason for the intervention, how to perform it safely and accurately, and the assessment needs pre- and post-intervention. For example, to administer pain medications as an intervention, the nurse must first assess the patient pain scale using a preapproved tool specific to their care environment. If the tool's results are analyzed by the nurse and warrant pain medication (e.g., a 7/10 pain report), the nurse can administer the pain medication and check whether it was effective at a measured time (typically one hour after intervention). In almost all aspects of the implementation phase, some level of assessment (pre-, during, and/or post-intervention) is essential.

Evaluation

The final step of the nursing process is the *evaluation* phase. During this phase, the nurse evaluates whether the treatment plan (including all steps of the nursing process previously completed) was successful in meeting the patient outcome goals. If a goal has been met, based on measurable standards set, this diagnosis/outcome/goal can be considered "complete" and may be removed from the patient care plan. If a goal is not met or only partially met, however, the nurse must use critical thinking to analyze potential reasons for this failure. This process may include reassessing the patient, redesigning or modifying interventions and/or goals, searching for errors within the design or implementation of the care plan, and/or reevaluating the patient's individual situation and needs (Potter et al., 2017).

Given that evaluation is a form of assessment, many of the same tools used for patient assessment may be involved in the evaluation phase (Potter et al., 2017). For example, you may be physically assessing an area of the body to look for improvement in a surgical incision or an injury. Or, a rating scale of some sort (pain scale, fall risk scale, etc.) may be readministered after the implementation phase to see if goals and outcomes were effectively met. It is the nurse's responsibility to set up the parameters that will be used for the evaluation step, all of which should be evidence-based and readily available to any member of the nursing care team.

Conclusion

The nursing process is designed to guide nurses in a universal, stepwise fashion so that they can provide meaningful, effective, safe, and patient-centered care regardless of the point-of-care time or setting. Nurses and nursing students should be extensively familiar with all aspects of the nursing process to ensure they are delivering appropriate care to the patients they are serving.

REFERENCES

Chiffi, D., & Zanotti, R. (2014). Medical and nursing diagnoses: A critical comparison. *Journal of Evaluation in Clinical Practice, 21*(1), 1–6. https://doi.org/10.1111/jep.12146

Herdman, T. H., Kamitsuru, S., & Lopes, C. (Eds.). (2021). *NANDA international nursing diagnoses: Definitions & classification, 2021–2023* (12th ed.). https://shop.thieme.com/nanda-international-nursing-diagnoses/9781684204540

Nurjannah, I., Warsini, S., & Mills, J. (2013). Comparing methods of diagnostic reasoning in nursing. *GSTF Journal of Nursing and Health Care, 1*(1).

Potter, P. A., Perry, A. G., Stockert, P. A., & Hall, A. (2017). *Fundamentals of nursing* (9th ed.). Elsevier.

Toney-Butler, T. J., & Thayer, J. M. (2023, April 10). Nursing process. *StatPearls.* https://www.ncbi.nlm.nih.gov/books/NBK499937/

CHAPTER 3

Answering NCLEX-Style Questions

Andrea Adimando, DNP, MSN, MS, APRN, PMHNP-BC, BCIM

Introduction

As discussed briefly in Chapter 1, The National Council Licensure Examination (NCLEX) is the nationwide licensure examination used in the United States. The NCLEX is developed and administered by the National Council of State Boards of Nursing (NCSBN). Once you graduate from your nursing program, you are required to meet the minimum passing requirements of the NCLEX before you can apply for state licensure. The exam ensures that you are competent to enter professional practice as an entry-level nurse.

In April 2023 a new model of the NCLEX, the "Next Generation (Next-Gen) NCLEX," was deployed. The NextGen NCLEX contains some new styles of multimodal questions that will be described and explained

The Appendix of this book contains a series of "NCLEX-style" questions for several of the chapters and topics that have been covered. Although you may wish to try and answer some of these questions to test your knowledge prior to completing the chapters, it is strongly recommended that you attempt these questions after you have completed the case study exercises within each chapter to test your retention and ability to apply the material you have learned and practiced.

within this chapter. NextGen also contains unfolding case studies with questions embedded within to gauge the nurse's ability to apply critical thinking, prioritizing, and complex decision-making within a realistic patient care scenario. One case study may have several items that follow to assess the nurse's clinical decision-making skills.

This chapter guides you through a stepwise process for answering NCLEX-style questions, including NextGen-style questions, giving you examples, tips, and strategies that may be useful to you as a set of tools for answering these questions throughout your nursing school program and for the NCLEX itself. Because the NCLEX is ever-changing, we strongly recommend that you review the most recent NCLEX test plan prior to taking the exam to ensure you have a good idea of the current layout, content, and structure of the exam.

The Anatomy of NCLEX Questions

Prior to NextGen, there were five styles of NCLEX questions:

1. Multiple choice
2. Multiple response
3. Hotspot
4. Fill-in-the-blank
5. Drag-and-drop/ordered response

The following sections explore these five styles with a sample question and explanation.

Multiple Choice Question

The first, and most popular, is the multiple-choice question. This format presents the test taker with a stem and then four potential responses with only *one* correct answer possible. For example:

SAMPLE QUESTION 1

While taking a walk, Mr. Jones notices the sky appears dark and stormy. This seems odd considering the sky is normally:

A) Red   **C)** Blue

B) Green   **D)** Orange

Answer: C

RATIONALE
In the example above, the correct answer is obviously "C" or "Blue." Multiple choice questions on the NCLEX can be written to evaluate simple recall of information, or they can be more complex scenarios to evaluate analysis and application.

Multiple Response Question

Another question style found on the NCLEX includes multiple response questions (often referred to as "select all that apply" questions), in which the stem of the questions asks the test taker to identify *all* correct answer choices. For example:

SAMPLE QUESTION 2

When looking outside, the nurse recognizes that all of the following are green: *(Select all that apply)*

A) Leaves

B) Grass

C) Sky

D) Clouds

Answer: A and B

RATIONALE

In the example above, "A" and "B" would be the correct choices. In this style of question, no partial credit is given. You must correctly identify *all* correct responses to receive credit for the question. Some find this style of question to be more challenging because the exam does not indicate the number of correct responses. Though not common, it is possible for a multiple response question to only have one correct answer, or for all given answer choices to be correct. Typically, several pieces of knowledge are required to answer questions of this type, contributing to their difficulty level.

The remaining three styles of questions you may encounter on the NCLEX are also known as *alternate format questions*. Though you are less likely to encounter alternate format questions than multiple choice or multiple response, you should still be prepared to answer alternate formats. Types of alternate format questions include hotspot, fill-in-the-blank, and drag-and-drop or ordered response questions.

Hotspot Question

Hotspot questions present test takers with an image and ask them to identify a specified region or element. For example:

SAMPLE QUESTION 3

Click on the image that would signal a driver to stop:

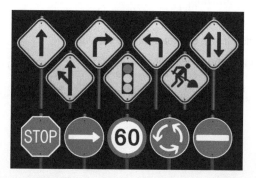

In nursing, this may equate to an image of a body part where the nurse needs to click the area that is to be assessed, such as the areas of auscultation of the heart. Further examples will be given at the end of this chapter.

Fill-in-the-Blank Question

Fill-in-the-blank questions provide the test taker with an open prompt within the stem. This style of question requires you to correctly complete a statement by inserting a word, phrase, or numeric value to make the statement true. The question may have a single fillable space or multiple. For example:

SAMPLE QUESTION 4

A _____ will bark while a _____ will meow.

To correctly complete the sentence, the test taker would type the word "dog" in the first space and "cat" in the second. Responses for this style of question are entirely generated by the test taker; there is no word bank provided. In the same manner as the multiple response questions, credit will only be given if each required space receives a correct response. In nursing, these will sometimes include calculations, where the test taker is required to enter a numerical value in the blank (such as a medication calculation, IV drip rate, etc.).

Drag-and-Drop Question

The final question type is the drag-and-drop or ordered response question. This question asks the test taker to order or prioritize pieces of information. This might include placing the steps for a procedure in the correct order or appropriately prioritizing steps of the nursing process. For example:

SAMPLE QUESTION 5

When mopping a floor, the correct sequence of actions is:

    A) Rinse and dry the mop.

    B) Fill the bucket with water.

    C) Place the mop in the bucket until it is saturated.

    D) Use the mop to mop the floor.

Answer: B, C, D, A (in that order)

RATIONALE

In this example, the proper sequence would be B→C→D→A, which the test taker would indicate by dragging the answer choices and placing them in the correct order. In nursing, these questions typically encompass material on prioritizing patient care according to the symptoms a patient or group of patients is manifesting. Later in the chapter we discuss strategies for prioritization using concepts such as the nursing process and the "ABC" rule.

There may also be audio questions, in which test takers are required to listen to something (perhaps a breath sound, heart sound, bowel sound, etc.) and answer a question based on what they heard. While these questions are generally uncommon, they may potentially make an appearance on your NCLEX-RN exam.

New Styles of Questions in the NextGen NCLEX

The NextGen exam has added the following four types of questions:

1. Extended multiple response
2. Case studies
3. Stand-alone
4. Bowtie

Extended Multiple Response

Extended multiple response questions are similar to the "select all that apply" questions mentioned above, but the NextGen multiple response questions may have up to 10 answer choices available to the test taker. Points are given for correct responses and removed for incorrect responses. See the exemplar in the second case study below.

Case Studies

Case study items (see samples in Figures 3.1 and 3.2) are characterized by the following:

1. They contain clinical information for one or more clients.
2. They contain a group of six items that represents the clinical judgment model of NextGen.
3. They require the entry-level nurse to make multiple clinical decisions throughout the spectrum of the clinical judgment model.
4. They use an action-model approach by combining individual components in a structured format.

Sample Case Studies: NextGen Items

Case Summary:

A 78-year-old female is admitted with difficulty breathing. She reports shortness of breath when moving, sleeping, and resting. She states that she has been sleeping on a recliner with a pillow behind her head for the past week. She has a history of hypertension, atrial fibrillation two years ago, and appendectomy five years ago. The patient is being transferred to a cardiac telemetry unit for ongoing monitoring.

Nursing Notes	Vital Signs

1100: Patient arrived to room, alert and oriented x 3, shortness of breath noted with rest and with activity. Worsened with excessive talking.

Weight: 160lbs., BMI 24.5.

Cardiac: Monitoring initiated, sinus tachycardia noted. S3 noted on auscultation.

Respiratory: Increased work of breathing noted with activity, when talking, and when at rest. Crackles noted bilaterally throughout lungs, worsened in lower lobes.

18 gauge IV in left AC area. Orders received on arrival. Labs drawn, chest X-ray and echocardiogram ordered, results pending.

FIGURE 3.1 NextGen case summary question: Example 1.

SAMPLE QUESTION 6 (Multiple choice)

Based on the nursing notes in the electronic health record above, which would be the next most appropriate assessment?

A) Full set of vital signs

B) Pulmonary function test

C) Hemoccult

D) Urine dipstick

Answer: A

RATIONALE

A full set of vital signs is essential to the assessment and monitoring of this patient and to determine next steps.

In the case study format, additional information is given regarding the same case and another NextGen-style question will follow, such as in the example below.

Case Summary:

A 78-year-old female is admitted with difficulty breathing. She reports shortness of breath when moving, sleeping, and resting. She states that she has been sleeping on a recliner with a pillow behind her head for the past week. She has a history of hypertension, atrial fibrillation two years ago, and appendectomy five years ago. The patient is being transferred to a cardiac telemetry unit for ongoing monitoring.

Nursing Notes	Vital Signs

Time: 1105

Heart Rate: 110
Blood Pressure: 174/94
Oxygen Saturation: 93% on 3L Nasal Cannula
Respiratory Rate: 28
Temperature: 98.4
Pain: 1/10

FIGURE 3.2 NextGen case summary question: Example 2.

SAMPLE QUESTION 7 (Multiple response)

Based on the vital signs in the electronic health record above, which findings are significant and require follow-up? *(Select all that apply)*

☐ Shortness of breath with activity/talking
☐ Respiratory rate 28
☐ Temperature 98.4
☐ Pain 1/10
☐ Blood pressure 174/94
☐ Oxygen saturation 93% on 3L Nasal Cannula
☐ Heart rate 110
☐ Sinus tachycardia
☐ Weight 160 lbs.
☐ BMI 24.5
☐ S3 noted

Answer: Shortness of breath, Respiratory rate 28, BP 174/94, Heart rate 110, Sinus tachycardia, S3 noted

RATIONALE

The above is an example of an extended multiple response, one of the new NextGen question formats, as it contains more than five answer choices for a "select all that apply" question.

A set of case study questions will continue providing additional information to the reader with each of the remaining questions that follow (usually a total of six questions per case study). One or more of the question formats described within this chapter may be utilized for each of the case study questions.

Stand-alone

Stand-alone items remain on the NextGen NCLEX in addition to case study items. Stand-alone items differ from case study items in that stand-alone items:

1. Have a stated diagnosis or an implied diagnosis
2. Include clinical information for one specific client
3. Generally require the entry-level nurse to make one, not multiple, clinical decisions

Note: Case study and stand-alone items may contain elements of any of the NCLEX-style question types listed within this chapter.

Bowtie

Bowtie items assess all aspects of the clinical judgment model within the same question. According to NCSBN:

> Bowtie items address all six steps of the NCJMM [NCSBN Clinical Judgment Measurement Model] in one item. The entry-level nurse has to read the scenario on the left to recognize if findings are normal or abnormal (Recognize Cues), understand the possible complications or medical conditions the client may be experiencing (Analyze Cues), and identify possible solutions to address the client's needs and issues (Generate Solutions). The entry-level nurse will then answer the bowtie item on the right to determine the most likely cause of the client's issues (Prioritize Hypotheses), the appropriate actions to take (Take Action), and the parameters to monitor once interventions have been implemented (Evaluate Outcomes). This is why it is called a "bowtie" item—because the response area looks like a bowtie with two "Actions to Take" on the left, two "Parameters to Monitor" on the right, and a single "Potential Condition" response in the middle. (NCSBN, 2021, p. 2)

Bowtie items provide the nurse with a series of tabs, typically resembling an electronic health record patient entry, that give the reader a variety of information on a patient to answer the question that is posed. These tabs may include headings such as "Nurses' Notes," "History and Physical," "Laboratory Results," "Vital Signs," "Admission Notes," "Intake and Output," "Progress Notes," "Medications," "Diagnostic Results," and "Flow Sheet."

Figure 3.3 shows a sample bowtie item. Notice the tabs that are provided to the nurse and the tokens given as options to deposit into the target boxes.

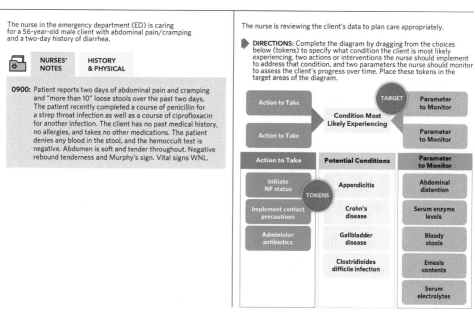

FIGURE 3.3 Bowtie question format. *Adapted from NCSBN, 2021.*

SAMPLE QUESTION 8

Follow the directions in Figure 3.3 to complete the diagram.

ANSWER/RATIONALE

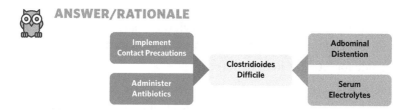

Given that the patient reported a recent history of multiple antibiotic use and is currently presenting with abdominal pain/tenderness, a negative Murphy's sign (gallbladder disease), and a negative rebound tenderness test (for appendicitis), this is most likely clostridioides difficile (C. diff). We want to monitor for peritonitis, which would be evidenced by abdominal distention, as well as serum electrolytes due to the patient losing fluids because of dehydration. The interventions listed would be appropriate for a suspicion of C. diff infection.

If a student chooses one incorrect answer in one of the bowtie answer boxes, they would be given partial credit for this item.

What Makes an NCLEX-Style Question Unique?

NCLEX-style questions are generally worded in a way that requires analysis and interpretation before you even attempt to answer. Questions are known for providing more information than necessary, requiring the test taker to discern what is relevant and what is not. A question stem may prompt you to select an option that is *not* correct or *most* correct, and if you miss those key differentiating terms while taking the exam, you will likely select the wrong answer.

It is also a possibility for a multiple choice question to have more than one correct answer. The challenge is to choose which item is most correct based on the stem of the question. These nuances may prove challenging for a test taker who is unfamiliar with the NCLEX format.

Nursing programs are aware of the learning curve associated with correctly interpreting and answering NCLEX-style questions, which is why many of your nursing exams will be constructed to reflect this format. Including NCLEX-style questions as part of your study routine will likely improve your performance as a nursing student and better prepare you for the certification exam.

NCLEX Test Plan

The NCLEX test plan is used for two purposes:

1. As a guide for test takers to give an overview of topics covered as well as the degree of their coverage to aid in exam preparation
2. As a guide for NCLEX item writers

The test plan is revised and republished every three years, ensuring that content is aligned with current practice and existing nurse practice acts. The newest test plan was effective as of April 2023 (NCSBN, 2022) and therefore will be the test plan that is discussed within this chapter.

The NCLEX test plan structure is devised to be in line with the contents of the NCLEX examination to provide a guide for educators and students when preparing for this examination. Figure 3.4 illustrates the NCLEX-RN test plan.

DISTRIBUTION OF CONTENT FOR THE NCLEX-RN TEST PLAN

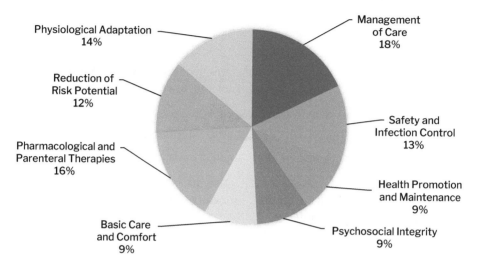

FIGURE 3.4 NCLEX-RN test plan (NCSBN, 2022).

The Client Needs Framework

The NextGen NCLEX is structured using the "client needs" framework "because it provides a universal structure for defining nursing actions and competencies and focuses on clients in all settings" (NCSBN, 2022, p. 7). *Client needs* is a concept that is divided into four major categories and further into subcategories. These are (NCSBN, 2022, p. 9):

- Safe and effective care environment
  - Management of care
  - Safety and infection control
- Health promotion and maintenance
- Psychosocial integrity
- Physiological integrity
  - Basic care and comfort
  - Pharmacological and parenteral therapies
  - Reduction of risk potential
  - Physiological adaption

> Given that the NCLEX is *adaptive* in nature, meaning its contents will fluctuate slightly based on the test taker's ability (discussed in more detail later in this chapter), the content quantity displayed in Figure 3.4 may differ by +/- 3% for an individual test taker.

Additional NCLEX Categories

In addition to the major categories of client needs, the NCLEX-RN also integrates concepts from nursing prerequisite coursework, including:

- Social sciences such as psychology
- Biological sciences such as anatomy & physiology and microbiology
- Physical sciences such as physics and chemistry

Additional important nursing concepts that are interwoven within the client need categories and will be important for you to have mastered prior to entering the examination include:

- The nursing process
- Caring
- Communication and documentation
- Teaching and learning
- Culture and spirituality
- Clinical judgment

Clinical judgment is a new addition to the NextGen NCLEX and may be posed as a case study or as an individual item. Case studies, also new to Next-Gen, contain six items that correlate with one client presentation, share client information in an unfolding manner, and address the following components of clinical judgment (NCSBN, 2022, p. 4):

Recognize cues: Identify relevant and important information from different sources (e.g., medical history, vital signs).

Analyze cues: Organize and connect the recognized cues to the client's clinical presentation.

Prioritize hypotheses: Evaluate and prioritize hypotheses (urgency, likelihood, risk, difficulty, time constraints, etc.).

Generate solutions: Identify expected outcomes and use hypotheses to define a set of interventions for the expected outcomes.

Take action: Implement the solutions that address the highest priority.

Evaluate outcomes: Compare observed outcomes to expected outcomes.

Techniques for Mastering NCLEX-Style Questions

One of the major differences between the NCLEX-RN and other certification exams is that there may be more than one correct answer to the question. Often the test taker is tasked with selecting the "best" answer (or answers, if a "select all that apply" question) from a series of options. Here is a series of techniques you can utilize when answering any type of NCLEX question, including those that require you to choose the best out of a series of options.

 Many test takers feel overwhelmed when they initially are introduced to NCLEX-style questions, ideally in the beginning of their nursing programs. This is normal, and it should be embraced as an opportunity for learning and practice rather than feared or avoided. NCLEX-style questions are highly complex and often involve a new way of thinking and synthesizing multiple levels of information.

Read the Question Very Carefully and Thoughtfully

Although this may sound silly and obvious, many students do not fully read the stem of the question.

The *stem* is the text body of the question that lets readers know what is being asked of them and presents all the information they need to answer the question.

Before jumping to the answer choices, which may result in an impulsive or ill-informed selection of the answer, it is important to ask yourself before and after reading the question stem (and before looking at the answer choices!):

- What is this question really asking of me?

  Is it asking you to simply recall and regurgitate knowledge, apply a concept, or prioritize nursing interventions? Is it asking you to act according to the nursing process?

- What information do I need to answer this question?

  This may include information that is being given to you in the question stem (e.g., a lab value, an assessment finding, a patient complaint, etc.) or information that you have learned throughout your nursing program (e.g., normal range of lab values, the nursing process, etc.).

- Have I read into this question and added factors that are not important or not valid?

  Often, exam takers will make a question harder than it actually is by assuming information that was not in fact given, or making a patient sicker than they really are by overthinking the question. Be sure you are not doing this before you move on to looking at the answer choices, as this will help you be less likely to choose the distractors that may be geared toward "overthinkers."

Here is an example of a question to which you can apply these principles:

QUESTION 3.1

Clients with coronary artery disease (CAD) go through several stages before becoming severely compromised. In considering the pathophysiology of CAD, the nurse would identify what physical response that does not occur in the early stages of CAD?

A) Decreased urine output

B) Dyspnea on exercise

C) Anginal pain relieved by rest

D) Increased serum triglyceride levels

(Zerwekh, 2016, p. 10)

Answer: A

 RATIONALE

Using the three strategies described above, let's analyze the stem:

- What is this question really asking of me?

  The question is asking you to identify what is *not* a characteristic finding in the early stages of CAD. In reading the stem, you can tease this out by the phrase "early stages of CAD" and "does not occur." The question cannot be answered correctly without understanding this.

- What information do I need to answer this question?

  The information needed to answer this question is symptoms of early-stage CAD and symptoms of late-stage CAD. Both would be pre-existing knowledge pieces you would have gleaned from your nursing school education. There is no patient-related information given to you in this question.

- Have I read into this question and added factors that are not important or not valid?

  The only pieces of knowledge and/or information you need to answer these questions are mentioned immediately above—the symptoms of the stages of CAD. Since there is no particular patient given as an example here, you do not need to individualize this answer to any particular patient. Be sure you are not adding any "what ifs" such as, "But what if this patient also has XYZ condition that patients with CAD frequently have?" Stick with the facts that you have and the information you know from your pathophysiology.

The answer to the question is A: A decrease in urine output, as this would happen when cardiac output is severely decreased and renal perfusion is poor—both of which happen in late, not early, stages of CAD. All the other distractors happen in early-stage CAD.

Consider Your "ABCs"

The "ABCs," as frequently referred to in nursing school, are **A**irway, **B**reathing, and **C**irculation. The authors of this book would also like you to consider the "S" for **S**afety, after you have considered A, B, and C. Considering the ABCs may help you in priority-style questions that ask you to determine which would be your "next" or "immediate" or "priority" action—all common terms seen in question stems that are trying to glean this information from you. Each term is outlined in Table 3.1.

TABLE 3.1 The ABCs

Airway	Ensure the patient has a clear or "patent" (usable, functioning) airway.
Breathing	You need to be sure the patient is breathing adequately.
Circulation	You need to be sure your patient's blood is properly flowing, circulating, and perfusing their body.
Safety	Once you have established that the patient has a patent airway, is breathing adequately, and circulating, you should always consider their safety before moving on to other priorities or interventions.

Without these functions being intact, the patient cannot function or survive, so these are your priority assessments for all patients, *in this order.*

Identifying ABC-Style Questions

Terms that may be used to clue you in to the fact that this is a prioritizing question might include:

- Which of these patients should the nurse see first?
- A patient arrives back to the nurse's care after XYZ procedure...
- Which of these tasks should the nurse perform first?
- A patient arrives by ambulance...
- A patient was just admitted to the nurse's floor...

These are just some of the examples that you may see in a question stem that are directing you toward prioritizing assessments or care interventions for a particular patient (or group of patients). The following question requires knowledge of the ABCs.

QUESTION 3.2

A patient has just returned from a cardiac catheterization procedure. The patient has a pressure dressing on her right groin area and a patent IV in her right arm. She was given morphine for pain immediately before arriving back to your floor. Vital signs are:

Temperature 98.6°F, Radial Pulse 80, RR 18, SpO2 96% on room air.

Which of these is the priority nursing action?

A) Initiate IV fluids due to NPO status.

B) Check femoral and lower extremity pulses.

C) Initiate 1L O2 via nasal cannula.

D) Ensure side rails of bed are in place.

Answer: B

RATIONALE

A patient who has received a cardiac catheterization in the groin area will need to be assessed for circulation to the lower extremities, given that the femoral arteries/veins have been disrupted during the procedure and are responsible for perfusing this area of the body. We can come to this conclusion using our ABCs:

If you had trouble with this question, try reviewing the strategies/questions discussed in the previous section. Did you add any information that wasn't actually given to you? Some test takers may have been distracted by the distractors because several sounded reasonable; however, the true priority here can only be determined by ruling out the ABCs first.

Airway: The patient has a patent airway, given that there is no information in the stem to indicate otherwise, and their SpO2 is WNL (within normal limits).

Breathing: There is no information in the stem about the patient having any difficulty breathing, and the SpO2 is WNL. Answer choice C would not be correct because there is no indication that this patient needs oxygen supplementation at this time.

Circulation: This is our priority given that the first two are ruled out. The nurse needs to ensure that the patient is perfusing and blood is circulating adequately, especially given the nature of the procedure they just had as stated above.

Safety: While this is a priority for all patients, the side rails are not the priority here. Nor is this patient at any particular risk of falls in this exact moment that would make this be our priority intervention.

Answer choice A is not an immediate priority because the ABCs take priority over any other assessment or intervention.

Here is another example of a prioritizing question related to the ABCs:

QUESTION 3.3

A nurse has just gotten a report on her four patients. Which of these patients should the nurse see first?

A) The patient who is on fall precautions and is consistently attempting to get out of bed

B) A patient who just returned from a bronchoscopy procedure whose O2 saturation is 86% on room air upon arrival

C) A patient who is requesting pain medication for 5/10 pain on day four post-op

D) A patient who is complaining of discomfort with urination

Answer: B

 RATIONALE
Let's go through each answer choice individually:

Answer A: While this of course is a highly dangerous situation for the patient, who was already deemed at risk for falls, this is not the priority if there are any patients who have compromised ABCs. This is also something that another staff member, such as a nurse's aide, could assist with, so this task could be delegated if the nurse has a more urgent patient to assess or intervene.

Answer B: This is the priority patient and the correct answer. Just reading this answer choice alone, without any stem or patient information, should alert you to an emergent situation. An SpO2 of 86% is an abnormal vital sign and needs to be addressed immediately. This is especially important in a patient who just returned from a procedure in the respiratory area.

Answer C: While pain is always important to address, this is not the priority in comparison to the patient in answer choice B. Another nurse could assist the patient with pain while you are addressing the urgent situation, or the patient can wait. While a pain scale of 5/10 is uncomfortable for a patient and should be addressed as soon as possible, it is not the urgent priority.

Answer D: While this patient may be experiencing a physiological response to an underlying issue (UTI, prostatitis, or any number of issues), this is not the priority as it is not an urgent or emergent situation. Using the ABCs (even including safety), this patient does not fall into any of these categories, and their complaints can wait without potentially causing any major harm to the patient.

Now let's build on this question.

QUESTION 3.4

Upon walking into the patient's room described in answer choice B, the nurse immediately notes that he appears short of breath. Which would be the order of the nurse's next actions?

A) Leave the room to call a rapid response and/or the provider.

B) Apply O2 via nasal cannula according to standing orders and elevate the head of the patient's bed.

C) Assess the patient's pulse and BP.

D) Check the patient's orientation to person, place, and time.

Answer: B→A→C→D.

RATIONALE

The nurse would not want to immediately leave the room to call for assistance from other staff members and/or licensed independent practitioners until the patient's breathing issues were at least partially addressed. Applying O2 and elevating the bed would be appropriate interventions the nurse could quickly do before leaving the patient. The provider should indeed be notified and/or a rapid response team given the nature of the patient's symptoms. Given the ABCs, the nurse should then assess vital signs and other signs of circulation while awaiting help. The patient's orientation, while important, does not take priority in this situation.

Remember the Nursing Process

As you learned in Chapter 2, the nursing process is pivotal to nursing education and nursing practice. While it may seem purely theoretical when you initially start your nursing education, you will soon realize that it is practical and relevant—and can be applied to many different aspects of nursing care. One of the strategies for answering NCLEX questions involves applying and differentiating aspects of the nursing process.

As mentioned earlier in this chapter, many NCLEX questions require the nurse to prioritize patient care based on information given and prior knowledge obtained in nursing school. If a question does not directly relate to the ABCs, the nursing process may be the next best framework from which to formulate your answer.

To help you evaluate which stage of the nursing process a question is geared toward, the following are some general characteristics that questions may have, depending on which phase of the process they are alluding to:

1. **Assessment:** These typically will be questions that involve collecting, confirming, and communicating data about a patient's condition. Look for keywords that may be referring to an assessment technique or need. However, if it is an emergent situation, be sure to note whether an intervention might be warranted (remember your ABCs) prior to initiating or completing an assessment.

2. **Diagnosis:** This phase, also called *analysis*, involves interpreting data (collected during the assessment phase) and making clinical judgments based on this interpretation. These can be very challenging questions as a result of the higher-level thinking required to answer them.

3. **Outcomes and planning:** This phase involves determining the expected clinical outcomes for your patient and planning how you will care for this patient to achieve said outcomes. If you do not yet have your assessment data or your diagnostic clinical judgment, it is nearly impossible to approach this step. Questions that involve creating a plan of care, determining outcome goals, and prioritizing problems when planning care are likely referring to this phase of the process.

4. **Implementation:** These questions almost always involve a nursing action, typically geared toward meeting the goals of the patient care plan. Remember that these questions are looking for a nursing intervention or other implementation strategy and not a medical one (though medical ones make great distractors). Anything involving communicating and/or documenting these interventions would also fall under this question category.

5. **Evaluation:** Questions about this phase of the nursing process usually involve comparing actual outcomes for a patient to the anticipated outcomes and determining whether the patient has responded appropriately to the care in place. Sometimes the evaluation will lead to a change in implementation, so these types of questions may be closely linked.

The most important thing to remember is that the nursing process is an "order of operations," so to speak. That is, you must assess before you diagnose, plan before you implement, etc. So, if you see a prioritization or a "next step" type of question, ask yourself, "What phase of the nursing process is this testing?" If you have not fully assessed yet, you should not be choosing an answer that involves diagnosing or intervening, for example. Here is a question that highlights this notion:

QUESTION 3.5

A nurse is accepting the assignment of a 2-year-old child who was brought in from his daycare facility after sustaining a fall from a piece of furniture. The nurse notices that the child has bruises and burns on his arms in various stages of healing and is fearful of adults. What is the nurse's priority action?

A) Notify the supervisor and/or physician that this child may be a victim of abuse.

B) Complete a full head-to-toe assessment of the child.

C) Call the state's department of child protective services to report the incident and the findings.

D) Apply antibacterial ointment to the burns and ice to the bruises, especially the new ones, to prevent further swelling or infection.

Answer: B

RATIONALE

The nurse's priority action is to complete a full head-to-toe assessment of the child. The nurse has not finished fully assessing the child or the situation, and assessment is the first step of the nursing process. The initial information being given in the stem of the question does not help us to determine the severity or pervasiveness of the injuries, so a more comprehensive assessment must be completed to determine the immediate and less acute needs of the child in question. The other interventions may be completed subsequently, but they are not the priority actions at this time.

Avoid "Shiny" Distractors

Remember, distractors (or incorrect answer choices) are put there to deter you from choosing the correct answer. By "shiny" we mean the ones that look or sound really good, even though they may not have much to do with the actual intent of the question. For example, NCLEX test makers know that you will be thinking about your ABCs. Can you pick out the "shiny" distractor in the following example?

QUESTION 3.6

A patient has just returned to his room from the recovery room after a lumbar laminectomy and is in stable condition. In considering possible complications the client might experience in the next few hours, what nursing action is most important?

A) Monitor vital signs every four hours.

B) Assess breath sounds every two hours.

C) Evaluate every two hours for urinary retention.

D) Check when he last had a bowel movement.

(Adapted from Zerwekh, 2016)

Answer: C

RATIONALE

The "shiny" distractor in this case is answer choice B. Many test takers will be attracted to this distractor because it mentions breathing; however, when considering the most common and/or potential complications a patient might experience after a laminectomy, does this answer really fit what they are looking for? The answer is no.

Options A and D are possible options for the future but not at this point in the patient's trajectory. Vital signs should be done much more frequently than every four hours for a postoperative patient, and constipation is not an imminent need or issue that needs to be addressed, so this would not be the priority.

> Remember, there was nothing in the stem that gave you any indication that this patient has respiratory issues, nor that this would be a potential problem for this particular patient or for any patient having this procedure. Be sure not to just jump to the "shiny" distractor in questions like these.

Remember Maslow's Hierarchy of Needs

Another important conceptual framework that will undoubtedly show up on the NCLEX-RN is Maslow's hierarchy of needs theory. Essentially, it is a way to categorize patient needs in a prioritized fashion. The hierarchy within this theory is displayed in Figure 3.5.

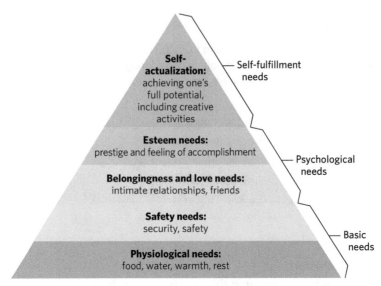

FIGURE 3.5 Maslow's hierarchy of needs.

With this theory, a person's physiological needs take precedence over all others. If their physiological needs are not met—basic things such as food, shelter, sleep—then the other needs cannot be adequately addressed. Therefore, when answering a question that may involve any level of patient need, Maslow's hierarchy should always be considered. If an answer choice addresses physiological needs, it is most likely the correct answer.

QUESTION 3.7

The nurse is caring for a pregnant patient with a deep vein thrombosis. The priority for the nurse is which of the following?

A) Providing explanations for the patient and her family members for all care procedures

B) Monitoring for changes in the physical condition of the mother and fetus

C) Reinforcement of DVT prevention strategies

D) Providing comfort measures for the patient

Answer: B

RATIONALE
Choice B is the only answer choice that addresses the physiological status and needs of the patient (and fetus). The others may be valid, but they are not priorities at this time.

Believe in Yourself!

You know more than you think you know. If you are finding it difficult to answer a question, bring yourself back to the strategies described above. If you are still coming up short, there are some tips and techniques to eliminate potential answer choices (distractors) to at least narrow your choices and increase your chances of getting the question right.

MORE STRATEGIES FOR SUCCESS

Evaluate key terms.

Many times, even if you do not know the answer to a question, or perhaps even what the question is asking, you can evaluate key terms within the stem that will lead you to which answer choice(s) might be potential answers. For example, if you see some of the prioritizing terms listed above, even if you do not know which answer choice is correct, you may be able to rank them in terms of priority interventions. If you are looking for an "immediate" or "next" priority, look for the answer choice that is a quick action or something that can be achieved relatively easily and quickly (i.e., placing a nasal cannula vs. implementing a long-term educational strategy for a patient). Eliminating any answer choices that may fit the longer-term category will help you prioritize your own answer choices and narrow them down.

Look for extremes.

Most answer choices that involve "extreme" words such as "never" or "always" are not the correct option. Eliminate any that contain these extreme terms to narrow down your answer choice field. The exception to this is if you are giving client education or providing a positive care technique. For example, telling a patient to "always check your blood sugar before administering short-acting insulin" is OK, as is a statement such as, "The nurse should always check patient identifiers before administering medication." There are almost never exceptions to these rules/policies, so they should not be considered "extreme."

Eliminate partially incorrect answer choices.

Sometimes answer choices are multifaceted and contain more than one piece of information or action. If even a small part of the answer choice is incorrect (or would never be correct), this answer choice should be eliminated from your options. A partially incorrect answer choice will never be the correct option, even if the other half is correct.

Look for a "correct but not now" answer choice.

There may be some distractors that sound good ("shiny") and might be correct in some circumstances, but ask yourself if they really answer the question at hand. For example, a question may ask what to do in case of an emergency. Forming a positive rapport with your patient is always going to be a good thing to do; however, in the

continues

case of an emergency, the nurse may not have time to do so and may need to implement an intervention or assessment before this is considered, so this would not be the correct answer.

Eliminate false security answer choices.

These are the types of responses by the nurse such as, "Everything will be all right," or, "You are going to get better really soon." These responses give patients a false sense of security, and the nurse or care provider who is making such claims cannot guarantee them. Therefore, any answer choice that sounds like this should be eliminated.

Avoid demanding or bossy responses.

These would be responses such as, "You really need to quit smoking for your health," or, "You should never do that." It is much better to provide the patient with motivational, therapeutic communication than to dictate what they should or shouldn't be doing.

Conclusion

The NCLEX-RN is an ever-evolving, complex examination with multiple facets and components. Given its complexity and importance to your nursing career, it is never too early to begin familiarizing yourself with the test plan and with NCLEX-style questions. Critical thinking, which is required to answer most NCLEX-style questions, is essential not only to passing this exam but also to your future nursing practice. It is our intention that this chapter remains a resource to you as you continue in your nursing studies and aids in your preparation for the NCLEX-RN.

REFERENCES

National Council of State Boards of Nursing. (2021). *Next Generation NCLEX news.* https://www.ncsbn.org/public-files/NGN_Spring21_Eng.pdf

National Council of State Boards of Nursing. (2022). *Next Generation NCLEX-RN® test plan.* https://www.ncsbn.org/public-files/2023_RN_Test%20Plan_English_FINAL.pdf

Zerwekh, J. (2016). *Illustrated study guide for the NCLEX-RN® exam.* Elsevier. https://pageburstls.elsevier.com/#/books/9780323280105/

CHAPTER 4

Introduction to Approaching the Patient Interview

Kristi Maynard, EdD, APRN, FNP-BC, CNE

The patient interview is often the first part of the physical assessment. The interview allows the nurse to collect subjective data from the patient about their health, past medical history, and any symptoms or complaints they are experiencing. The patient interview generally precedes the objective physical exam, and collected subjective information often guides the physical assessment. This chapter reviews the basics of performing a patient interview to help you in developing your own unique approach.

Getting Started

For most patient encounters, the interview will take place during your first meeting with the patient. This can be when a patient is being evaluated in the emergency department for an acute complaint or when they are presenting for their routine healthcare in an outpatient environment. The order and urgency of the interview may vary depending on the acuity of the patient and the care setting, but the steps are the same.

When you are preparing to interview a patient, understand that you are establishing a new relationship. How you approach your interactions with this individual will impact how receptive they are to answering your questions. Remember, you might be asking a stranger some very personal questions during the interview process, so establishing a relationship of transparency and respect is a critical step in the interview process. So how can you make a good first impression? There are some basic things you can do to assure your patient feels safe and comfortable in your care. First, do the best you can to make the interview environment private and comfortable. This might entail closing divider curtains, repositioning the patient if they are uncomfortable, or quieting noisy equipment like IV pumps or TVs. Ideally, you will position yourself in a manner that promotes conversation with the patient and reduces the feeling of inequitable power distribution. This means that you are at eye level rather than standing over the patient, you are facing the patient without obstruction, and you are focused on speaking directly to the patient and making eye contact rather than focusing your attention on a chart or computer screen. For example, you might consider pulling up a chair to the patient's bedside during the interview rather than standing at the computer.

Next, how you present yourself is important. Ensure you are professionally dressed and groomed. Introduce yourself and let the patient know what your role will be in their care. Then, ask the patient how they would like to be addressed. While some patients may feel more comfortable being addressed by their first names, others might prefer to be addressed more formally by their surname. Once you have established how the patient prefers to be addressed, it is a good opportunity to ask about your patient's preferred pronouns. Common gender pronouns include he, she, or they. Remember, a patient's pronouns are not the same as their sexual orientation, birth gender, or gender identity; this information can be evaluated separately.

Some of the questions that you will be asking may feel invasive to the patient. A good way to approach sensitive information is to ask kindly but directly and explain why this information is important to the patient's care delivery. Instead of making a patient feel guilty or awkward if they display hesitancy answering sensitive questions, reassure and support them to enhance trust and disclosure.

Asking Questions

The way you phrase questions will impact the patient response and the data you collect. You should strive to maintain a patient-centered focus when deciding how to phrase questions and how to respond to patient inquiry. Patient-centered care involves care delivery that focuses on the individual rather than the disease process. For example, we are not just asking questions about what diagnoses they have but also how those diagnoses have affected their activities of daily living.

There are two main question formats: open- and closed-ended questions. An *open-ended question* is formatted to allow the patient to provide a more detailed narrative response, while a *closed-ended question* usually requires a simple answer, like "yes" or "no." For example, when asking about the onset of a patient's pain, an open-ended approach would be, "Tell me about what you were doing when the pain began," while a closed-ended question might be, "Is it correct that you were running when the pain began?" There are times when one style of question might be more appropriate to use. In an emergency when you need to gather specific information quickly, the closed-ended approach is usually a better choice since you can ask direct questions quickly. On the other hand, the open-ended approach is more helpful when you are collecting a comprehensive patient health history.

Let's practice.

QUESTION 4.1 Open- and Closed-Ended Questions

Determine if the questions in this table are an example of open- or closed-ended questions:

Question	Open- or closed-ended?
"Were you born in 1986?"	
"Tell me about your surgical history."	
"What time did the pain begin?"	
"What are your current concerns regarding your health?"	

Answer: closed-ended, open-ended, closed-ended, open-ended

RATIONALE

Sometimes when collecting a response, you need to clarify the information the patient has provided. This step of the interviewing process allows you to confirm that you understood what the patient has told you and validates to the patient that you have been actively listening. You can do this by summarizing. Summarizing is when you repeat, in your own words, what the patient has told you. You may use phrases like "So I'm hearing you say" or "To summarize" to begin these statements. Using this method, if you have misunderstood something that the patient has told you, it gives them the opportunity to correct the information.

Focused Versus Comprehensive Interviewing

Depending on why the patient is seeking care, a focused or comprehensive approach to interviewing might be more appropriate. A focused interview focuses only on the details of the patient's presenting complaint and does not ask for information that is not relevant to why they are seeking care. As an example, if a patient was consulting with their primary care clinic because they suspected they had an ear infection, the nurse would not ask about a family history of cardiac disease. That is because a family history of cardiac disease would not impact the diagnosis or treatment of an ear infection. On the other hand, if a new patient is presenting to their primary care provider for an annual physical exam, the nurse would collect a comprehensive history because they need an inclusive picture of the patient's health. Deciding on whether to take a focused or comprehensive approach is often up to the nurse's judgment. Sometimes, nonspecific or vague symptoms necessitate a comprehensive history to look for details that may not be obviously related to the patient. For example, if the patient is presenting with fatigue, a comprehensive assessment might be performed because fatigue can be a symptom of many different conditions affecting most body systems. If a focused exam is performed, important information might be missed. Time may also be a factor when choosing your approach. In an urgent situation, a brief, focused exam might be more suitable than an extended, comprehensive interview.

Using PQRSTU to Aid in Data Collection

When collecting information about symptoms or a complaint, the PQRSTU mnemonic is a helpful tool to organize your questions. PQRSTU stands for:

P—Provoking/Palliative

This includes asking what makes the symptom better or worse.

Q—Quality

This looks to gather a description of the symptom.

R—Region/Radiation

This identifies the location of the symptom and whether other symptoms are associated with it.

S—Severity

This speaks to how severe the symptom is or how badly it is impacting the patient. We often see a 0–10 numeric scale used for this aspect.

T—Timing

This would include when the symptom started, how long it has been present, and also if it has ever been experienced before.

U—Understanding

This looks to capture the patient's perception of what is happening and can provide valuable insight into what the patient is experiencing.

Now, let's review some sample questions that would address each element of PQRSTU related to a complaint of chest pain.

QUESTION 4.2 PQRSTU

For each question, label it as the appropriate element:

Question	Element
How long ago did your chest pain begin?	
What do you think is going on?	
Can you tell me something that makes the pain feel better?	
Does the pain move anywhere other than the chest?	
On a scale from 0–10, how would you rate your pain right now?	
How would you describe your pain?	

Answer: T, U, P, R, S, Q

RATIONALE

P—"Can you tell me something that makes the pain feel better?" This question best addresses this element because it is asking the patient to identify anything that improves their pain, which can be referred to as a **P**alliative treatment.

Q— "How would you describe your pain?" In this question, the nurse is asking the patient to use descriptive terms to explain the features or **Q**ualities of their pain.

R—"Does the pain move anywhere other than the chest?" This question assesses if the pain is isolated to a specific region of the body or if it moves or **R**adiates.

S—"On a scale from 0–10, how would you rate your pain right now?" Using the pain scale allows the nurse to collect an objective measurement of the pain. This is a measurement method for determining the **S**everity.

T—"How long ago did your chest pain begin?" **T**iming can be addressed in a few ways using the PQRSTU mnemonic. In this example, the nurse is assessing when the pain first began. Other questions to address timing might include, "How long have you had the pain?" or "How often does the pain come and go?"

U—"What do you think is going on?" The nurse uses this question to gain insight into what the patient's perspective of their experience is. This can help us Understand what the patient thinks might be happening or provide more relevant information about the symptomology or patient history.

Common Pitfalls

Even the most seasoned nurse can fall victim to some of the common interviewing pitfalls. Being mindful and present during the interview process can help you avoid some of these practices that can otherwise impact the effectiveness of the patient interview.

First, be mindful of your body language. Body language is just as important as the spoken word when conveying your thoughts and emotions. This includes posturing, facial expression, and hand gestures. Standing in front of the patient with crossed arms may convey a closed-off or unapproachable demeanor, even if that isn't what you intend to deliver. Moderating your facial expressions is of critical importance. If a patient shares something that is surprising, even a slight raise of the brow can signal to them that you disapprove. Maintaining a pleasant, neutral expression is key.

We already discussed open- versus closed-ended questions, but just as important when constructing a question is avoiding wording that is leading or judgmental. For example, when asking a patient if they smoke cigarettes, a leading question would be, "You don't smoke, do you?" This gives the patient the impression that a response of "yes" would be unfavorable and might result in a dishonest response or lack of trust. Another example might be, "You had a rhinoplasty. Why would you do that?" which implies that the patient's decision to have the procedure was flawed and required explanation. Instead, remain factual and neutral when asking questions.

Be careful to avoid the use of jargon or technical language. *Jargon* refers to specialty words or phrases related to medical care. Often, phrases that we might use with medical peers because they are commonplace in our language can be difficult for patients to interpret. Instead, speak in layperson's terms when conversing with the patient to avoid confusion or miscommunication. An example would be using the term "stat." Instead of saying, "I'll be in to draw your blood stat," say, "I'll be in to draw your blood right away." Similarly, technical language can give the impression that you are trying to establish dominance or outsmart the patient. This would include using complicated or technical terms when common terms could be substituted. So instead of saying, "I'm going to lay you supine," say, "I'm going to lay you flat on your back."

A common pitfall when working with patients who are disabled, elderly, or adolescent is directing questions to their caregiver rather than the patient directly. This may be interpreted as a sign of disrespect to the patient and might hinder the development of the nurse/patient relationship. Instead, questions should be directed to the patients themselves using assistive techniques as needed to aid in communication, maintain eye contact, and take input from present caregivers as confirmed or acknowledged with the patient. In some cases, communicating directly with a caregiver is unavoidable, like with very small children or with adult patients who are severely impaired. If this is the case, be sure your communication with the caregiver is HIPAA-compliant, meaning you have written permission to speak with this person about the patient's health status. Also, make note in your charting that the primary source of data was not the patient but a caregiver, and note the nature of the relationship and the name of the person providing information.

Elements of the Patient Interview

When collecting patient data, you can approach the interview in a structured way to ensure all necessary information is collected. The usual progression of the interview is:

- Patient identifiers—name, date of birth, information source
- Chief complaint (CC)—This is the reason why the patient is seeking care.
- History of present illness (HPI)—This is a description of the events or circumstances of their presenting complaint.
- Past medical history (PMH)—This is a focused or comprehensive description of the patient's previous diagnoses and general health.
- Family history (FH)—This focused or comprehensive history will ideally include the patient's parents, grandparents, siblings, and children at a minimum. You may ask about a family history of a specific disease process or ask more generally about family diagnoses.
- Social history (SH)—This includes information about substance use, like tobacco, alcohol, or illicit substances; employment history; housing; relationship information; or sexual history.
- Review of systems (ROS)—The ROS, similarly to other aspects of the patient interview, can be focused or comprehensive. In a focused approach, you will only ask about pertinent symptoms related to body systems that are likely to be affected by the CC. In a comprehensive approach, all body systems would be addressed. The purpose of the ROS is to collect information on symptoms the patient might be experiencing to supplement information from the CC and HPI.

REVIEW OF SYSTEMS NARRATIVE SAMPLE

Constitutional: Denies fever, malaise, fatigue, loss of appetite, difficulty sleeping

Eyes: Denies vision changes, double or blurry vision

Cardiovascular: Denies chest tightness, pressure, pain, sensation of heart racing or skipping beats, or edema

Respiratory: Admits to shortness of breath, denies cough or trouble breathing

GI: Denies heartburn, acid reflux, or belching; negative for nausea, vomiting, diarrhea, constipation, abdominal pain, blood in stool, and stool changes

GU: Denies difficulty urinating, urinary frequency, urgency, incontinence, hematuria, painful urination, or changes in urination

Integumentary: Denies rashes, bruises, or new skin lesions

Neuro: Denies dizziness, lightheadedness, numbness, tingling, burning, or weakness in fingers, hands or arms

While it is your goal to move from one section to the next, sometimes it is unavoidable to move between sections during the interview. Learning to organize your interview and complete it in a timely fashion takes some practice. Finding a sequence that works for you is key!

Cultural Considerations

Each nurse should strive to deliver culturally competent care. Cultural competence requires sensitivity to a patient's heritage, sexual orientation, socioeconomic status, ethnicity, and cultural background (Cuellar et al., 2008). Part of being culturally competent is exercising cultural humility. *Cultural humility* is the ability to appraise and accept your own knowledge deficits and perspectives as they relate to others' cultures and cultural experiences. Building cultural humility is not an automatic process but instead is a purposeful process of self-reflection and continued education.

When delivering culturally competent care, there are a few things to consider during the interview. First, determine what the patient's primary or preferred language is. If you are not fluent in that language, you must secure a certified medical interpreter to facilitate your communication. It is important to use a trained medical interpreter rather than depend on a patient's friends and family because there are medical terms that may not translate directly, or information might be unintentionally miscommunicated, thereby impacting patient care. If a live medical interpreter is not available, language line services can be utilized to access thousands of languages within minutes.

When asking about language, be mindful not to use leading questions when determining language fluency. Asking a question like "You can understand English, right?" may make the patient feel uncomfortable identifying a different preferred language. Asking "What is your preferred language?" would be more appropriate.

Additional information that contributes to culturally competent care would include information about the patient's health beliefs. This may be impacted by their religion but may not be directly related, so be sure to ask about both. Health beliefs can include how the patient defines health and illness, what they feel influences wellness, and what they include as part of their personal health and wellness routines.

Certain cultures have preferences regarding the gender, age, or religion of the person caring for them. These requests should be accommodated to uphold the patient's cultural norms and beliefs whenever possible.

Emerging Technologies

Artificial intelligence, or AI, is rapidly emerging in the healthcare arena as a cost-effective, accurate method of patient data collection and even care delivery. Early studies predict that the use of AI in healthcare will reduce errors, improve accessibility, improve patient safety, and reduce the cost of healthcare.

While most patient interviewing is still happening between healthcare professionals and patients, the use of AI for interviewing and health history collection is on the rise. AI technologies are becoming so sophisticated that they can perform a patient interview with the ability to ask appropriate follow-up questions based on patient response. The mannerisms and voice quality are often indistinguishable from a real person, making AI interviewing a great alternative for telehealth and phone interviewing in rural areas or for those areas with poor medical infrastructure.

AI algorithms can be programmed to identity gaps in data collection or even discrepancies within a patient record. This reduces mistakes from human error resulting from omission or oversight. Another use of AI in the interviewing process is the ability to formulate a preliminary differential diagnosis or a list of the most likely diagnoses, based on the patient's responses to data point items like the chief complaint, history of present illness, and review of systems when combined with data about the patient's risk factors from their social and family history. This AI-generated differential diagnosis can even provide a percent of certainty for each diagnosis, allowing medical professionals to further pursue the highest priority diagnoses.

It is undeniable that you will be using AI technology during your career as a nurse as technology continues to be developed for use in the medical industry. Staying up to date and aware of AI uses and capabilities is an important part of continuing education for safe and effective patient care.

REFERENCE

Cuellar, N. G., Brennan, A. M. W., Vito, K., & de Leon Siantz, M. L. (2008). Cultural competence in the undergraduate nursing curriculum. *Journal of Professional Nursing*, 24(3), 143–149.

CHAPTER 5

Vital Sign Assessment

Ashley Dobuzinsky, DNP, MSN, RN, CNEcl

Vital signs are an integral part of performing a nursing assessment. Vital signs can be performed quickly and yield valuable information about the hemodynamic status of the patient. A full set of vital signs includes blood pressure, pulse, respiratory rate, temperature, and oxygen saturation.

There are important nursing considerations in the technique of obtaining and interpreting vital signs. This chapter reviews basic techniques for obtaining a full set of vital signs with nursing considerations for the pediatric and adult populations and provides opportunities to apply this knowledge.

Blood Pressure

Blood pressure is the measurement of the force of blood against the arterial walls.

Clinical Significance

Routine measurement of blood pressure is important for identifying trends and assessing for hypertension or hypotension (Muntner et al., 2019). Nurses routinely assess blood pressure as an indicator of hemodynamic stability to evaluate the effectiveness of medications and various interventions. The equipment needed to obtain a noninvasive blood pressure reading is a sphygmomanometer and stethoscope.

Proper Technique

There are several important nursing considerations when obtaining a blood pressure reading to ensure accuracy in the measurement.

Cuff Size

Blood pressure cuffs come in different sizes to accommodate different ages and body types. It is very important to select the correct size of cuff before obtaining a blood pressure reading. A cuff that is too small will yield a falsely high blood pressure, and one too large will yield a falsely low blood pressure. To ensure an appropriate size of cuff is used, first examine the cuff. Most blood pressure cuffs have markings to delineate where the patient's arm should fit. As a general rule of thumb, the inflatable part (called the *bladder*) of the cuff should cover 75%–100% of the circumference of the patient's arm (Muntner et al., 2019). Additionally, the width of the cuff should cover two-thirds of the length of the upper arm (Potter et al., 2023; see Figure 5.1).

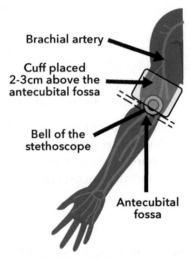

FIGURE 5.1 Cuff placement.

The blood pressure cuff should be placed around the upper arm, directly on the skin. Avoid rolling up sleeves or placing a cuff over clothing, as this can lead to inaccuracy in measurement. There should be a space of about 2–3 cm between the antecubital fossa and the bottom portion of the cuff (Muntner et al., 2019). Be cautious not to apply the cuff too loosely or too tightly. You should be able to fit two fingers in between the cuff and the patient's arm when it is secured correctly.

Patient Position

The ideal position for a patient to have their blood pressure measured is in the supine position with back support and feet flat on the floor (Potter et al., 2023). The patient's arm should be supported during blood pressure measurement and elevated to the level of the heart. The patient should avoid crossing their legs during blood pressure measurement, which can elevate blood pressure readings (Muntner et al., 2019; see Figure 5.2).

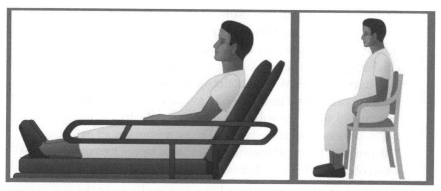

When on a bed or trolley, ensure the patient is sitting, with legs outstretched and uncrossed.

When seated, ensure the patient is in a chair with a backrest and positioned with feet on the floor and legs uncrossed.

FIGURE 5.2 Body position for taking accurate blood pressure readings.

Patient Considerations

Ideally, a patient should avoid ingestion of caffeine, exercise, and smoking in the 30 minutes prior to blood pressure measurement, as these activities can lead to elevations in blood pressure readings (Muntner et al., 2019). The patient should also empty their bladder prior to blood pressure measurement, as elevations of up to 10 mmHG have been observed among patients having a full bladder at the time of measurement (Sapra et al., 2023).

Avoid obtaining blood pressure measurements in the extremity of a patient who has an arteriovenous graft or fistula for hemodialysis, as this can affect patency of the graft or fistula (National Kidney Foundation, 2015). For patients who have had a mastectomy and/or an axillary lymph node dissection, consider avoiding blood pressure measurement in the affected arm, as this can potentially increase the risk for the development of lymphedema (American Cancer Society, 2021). Blood pressure measurement in the extremity of a peripherally inserted central catheter should be avoided, as well as in the extremity of a peripheral intravenous line while the patient is receiving intravenous infusions (Gorski et al., 2021). The extremity affected by acute deep vein thrombosis or injury/trauma should also be avoided.

Procedure

Before beginning with obtaining a blood pressure measurement, explain the procedure to the patient. Once you have determined the correct cuff size and the patient is positioned optimally, you can proceed with obtaining the blood pressure measurement.

1. To determine the patient's estimated blood pressure, place the blood pressure cuff on the patient's arm and palpate the brachial artery. Inflate the blood pressure cuff while simultaneously palpating the brachial artery and take note on the manometer when the pulse becomes no longer palpable. When obtaining the blood pressure, the blood pressure cuff should be inflated 30 mmHG higher than the measurement noted when the pulse was no longer palpable (Muntner et al., 2019). For example, if the brachial pulse was no longer palpable at 120 mmHG, the blood pressure cuff should be inflated to 150 mmHG when obtaining the blood pressure measurement.

2. To obtain an auscultatory blood pressure reading, put the cuff in place on the patient's upper arm and palpate the location of the brachial artery, then place the diaphragm of the stethoscope over the brachial artery.

3. Secure the dial on the manometer so that the cuff may be inflated, and then proceed with inflating the cuff to the estimated systolic measurement. Once the cuff is inflated, proceed with opening the dial on the air release valve slowly. The manometer should decrease by 2–3 mmHg per second to allow for accuracy in auscultation (Muntner et al., 2019).

4. The sounds that are heard when auscultating the blood pressure are referred to as *Korotkoff sounds.* The first audible sound is the systolic pressure. Continue to deflate the cuff by slowly releasing the air release valve and take note of the last sound heard—this is the diastolic pressure. The systolic and diastolic pressures are recorded in mmHg— for example, 110/70 mmHG.

See Tables 5.1 and 5.2 for normal and abnormal blood pressure measurements for adult and pediatric populations.

TABLE 5.1 **Adult Blood Pressure Measurements**

	Systolic Pressure		Diastolic Pressure
Hypotension	< 90		
Normal	< 120	and	< 80
Elevated blood pressure	120–129	and	< 80
Hypertension (Stage 1)	130–139	or	80–89
Hypertension (Stage 2)	> 140	or	> 90

(Whelton et al., 2018)

It is important to note that systolic pressures >180 and diastolic pressures >120 in the absence of symptoms such as chest or back discomfort or neurological changes are referred to as *hypertensive urgency* (American Heart Association, 2023b). Systolic pressures >180 and diastolic pressures >120 with symptoms of chest or back discomfort or neurological changes are referred to as *hypertensive crisis* and require immediate intervention (American Heart Association, 2023b).

TABLE 5.2 Pediatric Blood Pressure Measurements

	Systolic Pressure	Diastolic Pressure
Neonate	67–84	35–53
Infant	72–104	37–56
Toddler	86–106	42–83
Preschool age (3–5)	89–112	46–72
School age (6–9)	97–115	57–76
Preadolescent (10–12)	102–120	61–80
Adolescent (12–15)	110–131	64–83

(American Heart Association, 2020)

Among pediatric populations, the diagnosis of normal blood pressure is defined as systolic and diastolic pressures < 90th percentile when considering age, sex, and height percentiles (Flynn et al., 2017). High blood pressure is defined as systolic and diastolic pressures >/= 95th percentile when taking into account age, sex, and height percentiles (Flynn et al., 2017).

Pulse

Pulse, also referred to as *heart rate,* is the measurement of how many times the heart beats every minute.

Clinical Significance

Alterations in pulse can occur with a multitude of conditions. Establishing a baseline pulse rate allows the nurse to identify fluctuations in rate and rhythm and correlate the findings clinically.

The equipment needed to obtain a radial pulse is a watch with a second hand. The equipment needed to obtain an apical pulse is a stethoscope and a watch with a second hand.

Procedure

Before beginning with obtaining a pulse measurement, explain the procedure to the patient.

Pulses can be obtained in multiple places on the body; however, the most common places for obtaining a pulse measurement for vital signs is the radial artery or the apical pulse (Potter et al., 2023).

Radial Artery (Apical) Pulse Assessment

To obtain a radial pulse assessment, place your first two fingertips on the radial artery, located thumb side on the lateral aspect of the wrist. A grooved area between the radial bone and the tendon in the wrist is the most optimal location for obtaining the pulse (Potter et al., 2023; see Figure 5.3). Palpate for the radial artery until consistent pulsation is felt, and begin counting the pulsations for one full minute. The pulse is recorded in beats per minute (for example, 70 beats per minute).

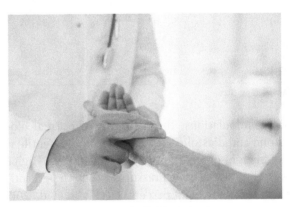

FIGURE 5.3 Radial/apical pulse.

To obtain an apical pulse, place the diaphragm of the stethoscope on the patient's chest along the fifth intercostal space at the left midclavicular line (Potter et al., 2023). This location is referred to as the *point of maximal impulse* (PMI) and is clinically significant because this is the point correlating to the location of the apex of the heart, where cardiac sounds are heard most prominently (Potter et al., 2023).

When the PMI landmark has been located, auscultate heart sounds, and when consistent S1 and S2 ("lub dub") sounds are heard, begin counting the heart rate for one full minute (see Figure 5.4).

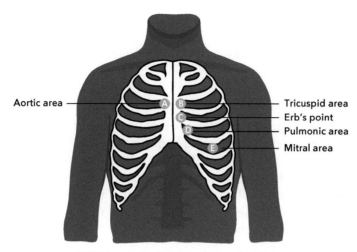

FIGURE 5.4 Cardiac auscultatory locations.

The apical pulse is recorded in beats per minute. Documentation should note that the pulse measurement was obtained apically. See Tables 5.3 and 5.4 for normal and abnormal pulse rates for adult and pediatric populations.

TABLE 5.3 Adult Pulse Rates

Normal	60–100 beats per minute
Bradycardic	< 60 beats per minute
Tachycardic	> 100 beats per minute

(American Heart Association, 2023a)

TABLE 5.4 Pediatric Pulse Rates

Neonatal	100–205
Infant	100–180
Toddler	98–140
Preschool	80–120
School age	75–118
Adolescent	60–100

(American Heart Association, 2020)

Respiratory Rate

Respiratory rate is the measurement of the number of breaths taken per minute.

Clinical Significance

Accuracy in measuring respiratory rate is critical because literature supports that alterations in respiratory rate are among the first signs that a patient's condition is deteriorating (Loughlin et al., 2018). Alterations in respiratory rate can occur in the setting of overwhelming infection, neurological disorders, anemia, and metabolic syndromes—and as side effects to certain medications (Hill & Annesley, 2020). The equipment needed to obtain a respiratory rate is a watch with a second hand.

Procedure

It is advisable to avoid acknowledging to the patient that you are counting their respirations because the patient may alter their respiratory pattern (Potter et al., 2023). To obtain a respiratory rate measurement, your patient should be lying or sitting comfortably so that visualization of chest rise and fall can occur unobstructed. To measure respiratory rate, each chest rise and fall is counted as one respiration. Respirations should be counted for one full minute. Avoid shortcut methods such as counting respirations for 30 seconds and multiplying the number of respirations by 2, as this can lead to inaccuracy in measurement, especially in patients with abnormal patterns of breathing (i.e., Cheyne-Stokes respirations). See Tables 5.5 and 5.6 for normal and abnormal respiratory rates for adult and pediatric populations.

TABLE 5.5 Adult Respiratory Rates

Normal	12–20 breaths per minute
Bradypnea	< 12 breaths per minute
Tachypnea	> 20 breaths per minute

(Hill & Annesley, 2020)

TABLE 5.6 Pediatric Respiratory Rates

Infant	30–53 breaths per minute
Toddler	22–37 breaths per minute
Preschool	20–28 breaths per minute
School age	18–25 breaths per minute
Adolescent	12–20 breaths per minute

(American Heart Association, 2020)

Temperature

Temperature refers to the measurement of the core body temperature.

Clinical Significance

Body temperature can be influenced by several factors, including age, environmental exposures, hormonal fluctuations, exercise, stress, and site of temperature measurement (Geneva et al., 2019; Potter et al., 2023). Routine temperature measurement can be valuable in the clinical setting for identifying a fever, which can indicate the potential presence of an infection.

Procedure

Following are the variations in the technique for obtaining a temperature measurement depending on the site chosen to obtain temperature and nursing considerations associated with each site.

Oral

Prior to obtaining the temperature, explain the procedure to the patient, and ensure that the patient has not had anything to eat or drink in the past 15 minutes, as this can affect the validity of the measurement. After explaining the procedure to the patient, power on the temperature device and place a disposable cover on the temperature probe. Instruct the patient to lift their tongue upward. Gently place the tip of the probe in the sublingual pocket, instructing the patient to lower their tongue and close their mouth. The thermometer should remain in place until the device alerts that the measurement is complete. Take note of the measurement for assessment and documentation purposes, and discard the disposable probe cover. See Figure 5.5.

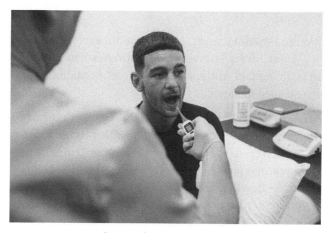

FIGURE 5.5 Proper placement of oral thermometer.

Axillary

If a patent is unable to tolerate an oral temperature or it is contraindicated, an axillary temperature can be obtained. Prior to obtaining the temperature, explain the procedure to the patient. Power on the temperature device and place a disposable cover on the temperature probe. Take note that the thermometer may require that the device is switched to axillary mode prior to obtaining the temperature (refer to manufacturer guidelines). Instruct or help the patient lift their arm upward, and place the temperature probe in the middle of the axilla. Instruct the patient to lower their arm and place their arm across their chest. The thermometer should remain in place until the device alerts that the measurement is complete. Take note of the measurement for assessment and documentation purposes, and discard the disposable probe cover. See Figure 5.6.

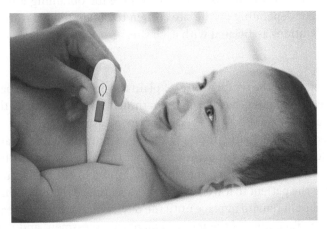

FIGURE 5.6 Proper placement of axillary thermometer.

Temporal

Depending on the manufacturer, temporal temperature probes can vary in functionality, from direct contact on the forehead to remote scanning in which there is no contact to the forehead. Refer to manufacturer guidelines on proper use of specific devices.

Prior to obtaining the temperature, explain the procedure to the patient. Ensure the patient's forehead is not moist, as this can influence temperature measurements (Potter et al., 2022). Power on the temperature device and place the temperature probe on the forehead (for direct contact devices). For remote contact devices, press the scanning button and begin sliding the temperature probe across the forehead in a linear fashion until the device alerts that the measurement is complete. Take note of the measurement for assessment and documentation purposes, and disinfect the device per manu-facturer guidelines. See Figure 5.7.

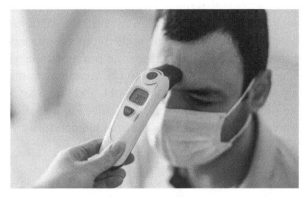

FIGURE 5.7 Proper method for obtaining temporal temperature.

Tympanic

Prior to obtaining the temperature, explain the procedure to the patient. Power on the temperature device and place a disposable cover on the probe. When inserting the thermometer into the ear canal, position the probe as closely to the tympanic membrane as possible. To achieve this in adults, pull the ear pinna backward, upward, and outward (Potter et al., 2022). In pediat-ric populations younger than 3 years of age, this can be achieved by pulling the pinna down and back (Potter et al., 2022). Among children older than 3 years of age, pull the pinna up and back (Potter et al., 2022). The device should remain in place until it alerts that the temperature measurement is complete. Take note of the temperature measurement for assessment and documenta-tion purposes, and discard the disposable probe cover. See Figure 5.8.

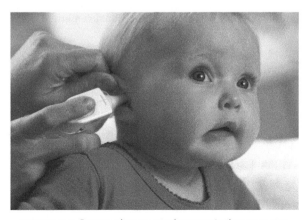

FIGURE 5.8 Proper placement of tympanic thermometer.

Rectal

Prior to obtaining the temperature, explain the procedure to the patient. Put on gloves to perform this temperature measurement. Assist the patient into a side-lying position with their leg drawn upward. Expose the patient minimally to promote privacy. Power on the temperature device, and place a disposable cover on the probe. Prepare the probe with lubricant prior to inserting the probe about 1.5 inches into the rectum for an adult patient, 0.5 inch for a pediatric patient < 6 months old, and 1 inch for > 6 months of age (American Academy of Pediatrics, 2020a). See Figure 5.9 for patient positioning and Table 5.7 for normal and abnormal temperature measurements.

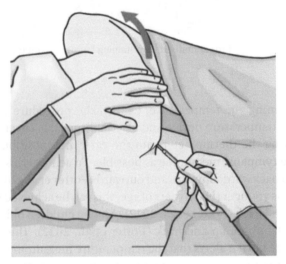

FIGURE 5.9 Proper patient positioning for obtaining rectal temperature.

TABLE 5.7 Adult and Pediatric Temperature Measurement

Normal (average)	98.6° F/37° C
Fever	>/ 100.4° F/38° C
Hypothermia	</ 95° F/35° C

(American Academy of Pediatrics, 2020a; Centers for Disease Control and Prevention, 2017)

Although the average normal temperature is 98.6°, a range of 97.7°–99.5° F is generally acceptable (Sapra et al., 2023).

Pulse Oximetry

Pulse oximetry (SpO2) is the noninvasive measurement of oxygen saturation in the blood.

Clinical Significance

Measurement of pulse oximetry requires the use of a device called an *oximeter*, which yields two light-emitting (LEDs), red and infrared light. When the device is clipped to the body, generally a fingertip, the lights pass through the body, and the absorption of these lights varies among blood that is oxygen-rich and blood that is oxygen-deficient. Oxygen-rich blood absorbs more infrared light, whereas oxygen-deficient blood allows more infrared light to pass through. The ratio of these two lights' absorption yields an estimation of the oxygen saturation of the blood, which is expressed as a percentage (Pesola & Sankari, 2023).

Procedure

To obtain an oxygen saturation measurement, place the oximeter on the part of the body that the device is indicated for use. Most pulse oximeters are designed to be placed on the fingertip. However, there are devices made specifically for earlobes, or adhesive bandage-style oximeters that can be taped to the finger or foot and are commonly used among pediatric populations. Ensure that placement of the oximeter is per manufacturer guidelines, as utilizing a device on an area of the body for which it is not intended can yield false measurements (Hlavin & Varty, 2022). Once the device is placed correctly, the device should be powered on, and the sensor should remain in place until a consistent waveform is established. Simultaneous assessment of the patient's radial pulse in comparison to the pulse measurement on the device can assist with checking accuracy. The measurement should be recorded as a percentage—for example, oxygen saturation of 98%.

Patient Considerations

There are several factors that can influence the accuracy of measuring an oxygen saturation, such as the presence of nail polish on fingernails, alterations in skin temperature, low perfusion states, and patient movement (Food and Drug Administration, 2021). Additionally, the evidence for racial bias among pulse oximetry—specifically, that devices yield overestimations of oxygen saturation and pose a patient safety risk in the identification of low oxygen states—has prompted a call for action among the medical community (Rathod et al., 2022). Awareness of this bias is critical for nurses and all healthcare providers who encounter situations where the accuracy of pulse oximetry measurements is in question, and this should prompt further analysis. Normal oxygen saturation for both adults and children is 95%–100% (Cleveland Clinic, 2022; Mau et al., 2005).

In assessing oxygen saturation values, take into account the patient's underlying conditions and baseline oxygen saturation levels. Patients with chronic respiratory conditions may have patient-specific acceptable oxygen levels that are lower than normal. Knowledge of these patient-specific criteria is critical when assessing oxygen saturation levels to determine if the level is acceptable.

Now that we have reviewed how to obtain a set of vital signs, let's apply this knowledge to an adult and pediatric case study.

 CASE STUDY 5.1

Patient Admitted to Medical/Surgical Unit With Gastrointestinal Bleeding

60-year-old male

Reports dark, tarry stools for one week

T 98.6° F	HR 104	BP 94/62	RR 22	O2 96%	Pain 2/10

Mr. Smith is a 60-year-old admitted to your medical/surgical unit today from the emergency department with a diagnosis of gastrointestinal bleeding. He reports dark, tarry stools for one week. Mr. Smith felt dizzy and nauseous today while at work, and a coworker drove him to the hospital.

While in the emergency department, Mr. Smith's initial blood work demonstrated an abnormal hemoglobin level of 7.7 gm/dL. Mr. Smith reports mild midabdominal discomfort and nausea. He reports a past medical history of hypertension and chronic back pain. He states that he has not taken his blood pressure medication for a few days because of the abdominal discomfort and nausea. The initial plan of care involves admitting the patient to the medical/surgical unit pending a gastroenterology consult in the morning.

QUESTION 5.1 (Multiple response)

Which of the vital signs above are most concerning? (*Select all that apply*)

A) Temperature
B) Heart rate
C) Blood pressure

D) Respiratory rate
E) Oxygen saturation
F) Pain level

Answer: B, C, D

RATIONALE

Mr. Smith's HR is 104 beats per minute, and a normal heart rate for adults is 60–100 beats per minute. Mr. Smith's heart rate is considered tachycardic. His blood pressure is 94/62 mmHG. Hypotension is typically defined as a systolic pressure < 90. While not critically low, a blood pressure of 94/62 in the setting of a patient with a history of hypertension who has not taken antihypertension medications and has gastrointestinal bleeding is concerning for hypovolemia. Mr. Smith's respiratory rate is 22, and a normal respiratory rate for an adult is between 12–20 breaths per minute. Mr. Smith's respiratory rate is considered tachypneic.

Gastrointestinal bleeding can result in a hypovolemic state, for which a low blood pressure might be expected. The compensatory mechanism for this loss of blood volume is the increasing of the heart rate. A blood loss of 15%–30% of the total blood volume will typically result in an increase in the heart rate for adults to 100–120 beats per minute and an increase in respiratory rate from 20–24 breaths per minute according to the hemorrhagic shock classification (Hooper & Armstrong, 2022). Mr. Smith's tachypnea can be explained by the loss of circulating blood volume, which has diminished the patient's oxygen-carrying capacity and therefore prompted the lungs to compensate by increasing the respiratory rate.

Patient information continued... During a routine nursing assessment, Mr. Smith tells you that he forgot to mention that he was recently started on aspirin by his cardiologist. While updating Mr. Smith's medication reconciliation record, he also reports that he takes nonsteroidal anti-inflammatory medications two to three times a day for back pain.

QUESTION 5.2 (Multiple choice)

Interpreting the relevant data, which of these four problems could have possibly occurred?

A) Mr. Smith has developed an infectious colitis from contaminated food.

B) Mr. Smith has developed gastrointestinal bleeding associated with concurrent use of NSAIDs and aspirin.

C) Mr. Smith has developed ischemic colitis.

D) Mr. Smith has experienced a myocardial infarction.

Answer: B

RATIONALE

It is possible that Mr. Smith has developed a gastrointestinal bleed associated with the frequent use of NSAIDs and concurrent use of aspirin. NSAIDs inhibit cyclooxygenase-1 (COX-1), which prohibits prostaglandins that serve to protect the gastric mucosa and can potentiate gastric irritation and bleeding (Ghlichloo & Gerriets, 2023). The development of infectious colitis has not been ruled out; however, Mr. Smith did not report symptoms typical of an infectious source (i.e., nausea, vomiting, and diarrhea). It is possible that Mr. Smith is suffering from ischemic colitis; however, this diagnosis would require further evaluation from the gastroenterologist.

Patient information continued... Mr. Smith presses his call bell, and you respond to the room and find him to be in acute distress. Mr. Smith has vomited a large volume of red blood and appears pale. He tells you he feels like he is going to "pass out."

QUESTION 5.3 (Multiple choice)

Based on this situation, what is the priority nursing intervention?

A) Call provider/initiate a rapid response team activation.

B) Obtain vital signs.

C) Establish IV access.

D) Administer scheduled medications.

Answer: A

RATIONALE

Mr. Smith is demonstrating signs of hemodynamic instability in the setting of acute hemorrhage. Summoning immediate assistance to the bedside of this patient is the priority. Vital signs can be obtained while awaiting the arrival of the provider or the rapid response team. Establishing IV access is important and can also be done while awaiting the arrival of the provider or the rapid response team. Administration of scheduled medications is not a priority because the patient is experiencing an acute change in condition. The appropriateness of medication administration during this situation can be established after the patient is evaluated by a provider.

QUESTION 5.4 (Multiple response)

Based on this situation, what orders would the nurse anticipate? *(Select all that apply)*

A) IV fluid resuscitation

B) Oxygen administration

C) Type and screen for ABO/compatibility

D) Obtain lab work (i.e., complete blood count)

E) Administer blood products

F) Prepare patient for transport to gastroenterology suite or surgery, if necessary

Answer: All of the above

RATIONALE

The nurse can anticipate that initial fluid resuscitation may be ordered pending administration of blood products for this patient, who may be acutely hypotensive in the setting of gastrointestinal hemorrhage. Oxygen administration should be anticipated because this patient has experienced acute blood loss and therefore has diminished oxygen-carrying capacity. Supplemental oxygen would be beneficial to prevent and/or treat hypoxia. Obtaining a type and screen for blood typing should be anticipated in the setting of acute hemorrhage if this was not completed prior to this acute event. Administration of blood products should be anticipated in the patient with acute blood loss and hemodynamic instability. Anticipating the transport of the patient to an interventional department or surgery for the treatment of acute hemorrhage is reasonable considering the need to identify the source of bleeding and intervene to stabilize the patient.

QUESTION 5.5 (Multiple response)

After implementing the plan of care, what findings would indicate that the patient's condition is improving?

A) BP 110/60   **C)** RR 24

B) HR 90   **D)** Persistent lethargy

Answer: A and B

RATIONALE

A blood pressure measurement of 110/60 is an improvement from the patient's initial blood pressure measurement of 94/62 mmHG. Similarly, an HR of 90 is an improvement from the patient's initial HR of 104 and demonstrates the patient's shift toward hemodynamic stability.

CASE STUDY 5.2

Patient Presents to Emergency Department With Fever

- 6-month-old female
- Parents report fever for three days, nasal congestion, and cough

T 102.4° F	HR 190	BP 74/46	RR 60	O2 95%

Mary is a 6-month-old female patient brought to the emergency department by her parents with a three-day history of fever, nasal congestion, and cough. Mary's parents report poor oral intake for three days. They report that Mary has no past medical history, and Mary was delivered at term.

The initial plan of care involves obtaining a complete blood count and electrolyte panel, performing a chest X-ray, and administering an antipyretic medication.

QUESTION 5.6 (Multiple response)

Which of the vital signs above are most concerning? *(Select all that apply)*

A) Temperature
B) Heart rate
C) Blood pressure
D) Respiratory rate
E) Oxygen saturation

Answer: A, B, D

RATIONALE

The threshold for fever is a temperature of >/= 100.4. Mary's temperature of 102.4 is considered a fever. Mary's heart rate is elevated and is considered tachycardic for her age. Mary's respiratory rate is elevated and considered tachypneic for her age. Mary's blood pressure is still within normal parameters for her age, and oxygen saturation is adequate.

Patient information continued...

Nurse's Note:

Mary is arousable to noxious stimuli but otherwise lethargic. Skin is pale, warm, and dry. Breathing is labored. Evidence of sternal retractions. Cough noted. Lungs with bilateral rhonchi. Abdomen is soft, nondistended, no observed pain response to light abdominal palpation.

Current Vital Signs:

T 101.9° F	HR 195	BP 72/40	RR 70	O2 89%

QUESTION 5.7 (Multiple choice)

You are concerned about the labored breathing, increased respiratory rate, and decreased oxygen saturation. What condition would most likely cause this presentation?

A) Urinary tract infection **C)** Upper respiratory tract infection

B) Pneumonia **D)** Otitis media

Answer: B

RATIONALE

While there are similarities in both the upper respiratory tract infection and pneumonia in that they can both produce fevers and respiratory symptoms, it is more common to have milder symptoms with an upper respiratory tract infection compared to pneumonia. In addition to fever, symptoms of pneumonia include cough, labored breathing, sternal retractions, and hypoxia, similar to the presentation of the patient in this scenario (American Academy of Pediatrics, 2020b). The option of a urinary tract infection is less likely given the lack of relevant data in this scenario to support this condition.

QUESTION 5.8 (Multiple choice)

Interpreting the clinical data and the most likely occurring condition, the patient is at high risk for:

A) Kidney failure **C)** Heart failure

B) Respiratory failure **D)** Skin breakdown

Answer: B

RATIONALE

The patient is exhibiting signs of respiratory distress/failure with an increase in respiratory rate, decrease in oxygen saturation, and evidence of increased work of breathing. There is no evidence in the relevant data to suggest the patient is in heart failure or kidney failure; therefore, the likelihood that these conditions are occurring, although not excluded, is low.

QUESTION 5.9 (Multiple response)

Based on this situation, what is the priority nursing intervention? *(Select all that apply)*

A) Notify provider of worsening condition.

B) Maintain patent airway/position patient to optimize breathing.

C) Provide supplemental oxygen as ordered.

D) Transfer patient to higher level of care.

Answer: A, B, and C

RATIONALE

Based on the acute deterioration of the patient, notifying the provider is a priority to summon immediate assistance to the bedside of the patient. Maintaining a patent airway by positioning the patient optimally (i.e., sitting patient upright) is a priority to allow for adequate ventilation. Administration of supplemental oxygen in the acutely hypoxic patient is reasonable pending advanced airway management. Transfer to higher level of care is likely to occur given the acuity of the patient; however, this is not the immediate priority. Stabilizing the patient prior to transport to higher level of care is the priority.

QUESTION 5.10 (Multiple response)

Based on this situation, what orders would the nurse anticipate?

A) Prepare for placement of advanced airway

B) Administer medications to facilitate intubation

C) Place patient on continuous pulse oximetry monitoring

D) All of the above

Answer: D

RATIONALE

The patient is demonstrating acute deterioration and signs of impending respiratory failure as evidenced by tachypnea, hypoxia, and increased work of breathing. It is reasonable to anticipate this patient may require an advanced airway and the need to prepare equipment to facilitate this intervention. The patient may require medications to facilitate intubation (i.e., sedative or paralytic medications), and the preparation of medications per provider orders should be anticipated. It is reasonable to anticipate placing the patient on continuous pulse oximetry monitoring to evaluate response to interventions.

REFERENCES

American Academy of Pediatrics. (2020a). *How to take your child's temperature.* https://www.healthychildren.org/English/health-issues/conditions/fever/Pages/How-to-Take-a-Childs-Temperature.aspx

American Academy of Pediatrics. (2020b). *Pneumonia.* https://publications.aap.org/pediatriccare/article-abstract/doi/10.1542/aap.ppcqr.396216/97/Pneumonia?redirectedFrom=fulltext

American Cancer Society. (2021). *For people at risk of lymphedema.* https://www.cancer.org/cancer/managing-cancer/side-effects/swelling/lymphedema/for-people-at-risk-of-lymphedema.html

American Heart Association (2020). *PALS digital reference cards.* https://shopcpr.heart.org/pals-digital-reference-card

American Heart Association. (2023a). *All about heart rate (pulse).* https://www.heart.org/en/health-topics/high-blood-pressure/the-facts-about-high-blood-pressure/all-about-heart-rate-pulse

American Heart Association. (2023b). *Hypertensive crisis: When you should call 911 for high blood pressure.* https://www.heart.org/en/health-topics/high-blood-pressure/understanding-blood-pressure-readings/hypertensive-crisis-when-you-should-call-911-for-high-blood-pressure

Centers for Disease Control and Prevention. (2017). *Definitions of symptoms for reportable illnesses.* https://www.cdc.gov/quarantine/air/reporting-deaths-illness/definitions-symptoms-reportable-illnesses.html#:~:text=CDC%20considers%20a%20person%20to,a%20history%20of%20feeling%20feverish

Cleveland Clinic. (2022). *Blood oxygen level.* https://my.clevelandclinic.org/health/diagnostics/22447-blood-oxygen-level

Flynn, J., Kaelber, D., Smith, C., Blowey, D., Carroll, A., Daniels, S., de Ferranti, S., Dionne, J., Falkner, B., Flinn, S., Gidding, S., Goodwin, C., Leu, M., Powers, M., Rea, C., Samuels, J., Simasek, M., Thaker, V., & Urbina, E. (2017). Clinical practice guideline for screening and management of high blood pressure in children and adolescents. *Pediatrics, 140*(3), 1–72. https://doi.org/10.1542/peds.2017-1904

Food and Drug Administration. (2021). *Pulse oximeter accuracy and limitations: FDA safety communication.* https://www.fda.gov/medical-devices/safety-communications/pulse-oximeter-accuracy-and-limitations-fda-safety-communication#:~:text=Follow%20your%20health%20care%20provider%27s,and%20use%20of%20fingernail%20polish

Geneva, I., Cuzzo, B., Fazili, T. & Javaid, W. (2019). Normal body temperature: A systematic review. *Open Forum Infectious Diseases, 6*(4), 1–7. https://doi.org/10.1093/ofid/ofz032

Ghlichloo, I., & Gerriets, V. (2023). Nonsteroidal anti-inflammatory drugs (NSAIDs). *StatPearls.* https://www.ncbi.nlm.nih.gov/books/NBK547742/

Gorski, L., Hadaway, L., Hagle, M., Broadhurst, D., Clare, S., Kleidon, T., Meyer, B., Nickel, B., Rowley, S., Sharpe, E., & Alexander. (2021). Infusion therapy standards of practice (8th ed). *Journal of Infusion Nursing, 44*(1). https://doi.org/10.1097/NAN.0000000000000396

Hill, B., & Annesley, S. (2020). Monitoring respiratory rate in adults. *British Journal of Nursing, 29*(1), 12–16. https://doi.org/10.12968/bjon.2020.29.1.12

Hlavin, D., & Varty, M. (2022). Improving patient safety by increasing staff knowledge of evidence-based pulse oximetry practices. *American Association of Critical Care Nurses, 42*(6), 1–6. https://aacnjournals.org/ccnonline/article/42/6/e1/31885/Improving-Patient-Safety-by-Increasing-Staff

Hooper, N., & Armstrong, T. J. (2022). Hemorrhagic shock. *StatPearls.* https://www.ncbi.nlm.nih.gov/books/NBK470382/

Loughlin, P. C., Sebat, F., & Kellett, J. G. (2018). Respiratory rate: The forgotten vital sign—make it count! *The Joint Commission Journal on Quality and Patient Safety, 44,* 494–499. https://doi.org/10.1016/j.jcjq.2018.04.014

Mau, M., Yamasato, K., & Yamamoto, L. (2005). Normal oxygen saturation values in pediatric patients. *Hawaii Medical Journal, 64,* 42–45. https://www.researchgate.net/profile/Loren-Yamamoto/publication/7866114_Normal_oxygen_saturation_values_in_pediatric_patients/links/56b2b60508ae5ec4ed4b59de/Normal-oxygen-saturation-values-in-pediatric-patients?_tp=eyJjb250ZXh0Ijp7ImZpcnN0UGFnZSI6InBlYmxpY2F0aW9uIiwicGFnZSI6InBlYmxpY2F0aW9uIn19

Muntner, P., Shimbo, D., Carey, R., Charleston, J., Gaillard, T., Misra, S., Myers, M., Ogedegbe, G., Schwartz, J., Townsend, R., Urbina, E., Viera, A., White, W., & Jackson, W. (2019). Measurement of blood pressure in humans: A scientific statement from the American Heart Association. *Hypertension, 73*(5), 35–66. https://www.ahajournals.org/doi/10.1161/HYP.0000000000000087

National Kidney Foundation. (2015). *Hemodialysis access.* https://www.kidney.org/atoz/content/hemoaccess

Pesola, G. R., & Sankari, A. (2023). Oxygenation status and pulse oximeter analysis. *StatPearls.* https://www.ncbi.nlm.nih.gov/books/NBK592401/

Potter, P., Perry, A., Stockert, P., & Hall, A. (2022). *Fundamentals of nursing* (11th ed.). Elsevier.

Rathod, M., Ross, H., & Franklin, D. (2022). Improving the accuracy and equity of pulse oximeters: Collaborative recommendations. *Journal of the American College of Cardiology, 1*(4). https://doi.org/10.1016/j.jacadv.2022.100118

Sapra, A., Malik, A., & Bhandari, P. (2023). Vital sign assessment. *StatPearls.* https://www.ncbi.nlm.nih.gov/books/NBK553213/

Whelton, P., Carey, R., Aronow, W., Casey, D., Collins, K., Dennison Himmelfarb, C., DePalma, S., Gidding, S., Jamerson, K., Jones, D., MacLaughlin, E., Muntner, P., Ovbiagele, B., Smith, S. C., Spencer, C. C., Stafford, R., Taler, S., Thomas, R., Williams, K., Williamson, J., & Wright, J. (2018). 2017 ACC/AHA/AAPA/ABC/ACPM/ AGS/APhA/ASH/ASPC/ NMA/PCNA guideline for the prevention, detection, evaluation, and management of high blood pressure in adults: A report of the American College of Cardiology/American Heart Association Task Force on Clinical Practice Guidelines. *Hypertension, 71*(6), e13–e115. https://www.ahajournals.org/doi/epub/10.1161/HYP.0000000000000065

CHAPTER 6

Assessing Mental Status

Dilice Robertson, DNP, MSN, APRN, PMHNP-BC, PMHCNS-BC

The mental status examination evaluates different areas of cognitive functioning and starts with observation, then moves to more internal functioning. The examination is an assessment of mental functioning by evaluation of general appearance, mood, all aspects of cognition, beliefs, and perceptions.

Observation

The mental status exam begins with observation—the elements that are assessed prior to an interaction with a patient—and then moves inward to more detailed observations elicited during the interview. Ensure privacy and a safe space for the conversation.

Active listening and empathy give the patient an opportunity to express feelings and thoughts without interruption. Showing genuine empathy and understanding by maintaining eye contact, nodding, and using supportive verbal cues like "I'm here to listen" or "I'm here to help you" allow for connection and investment in building therapeutic rapport.

The elements of the mental status exam are a collection of data points to assess for a change in functioning at a *snapshot in time*. The elements of the exam are identified in Table 6.1 with examples of findings within normal limits (typical) and the accompanying atypical findings. The findings are inferred and used to either corroborate or contradict other findings in a mental health assessment.

TABLE 6.1 Documentation of Observed Appearance

Element	Findings Within Normal Limits	Atypical Findings
Appearance (observation of the patient's age, dress, grooming, and hygiene)	Appears as stated age, dressed appropriately for the weather, clean, well groomed, good hygiene	Looks younger or older than stated age, not appropriately dressed for the weather, unkempt, disheveled, poor hygiene, malodorous, or poor dentition
Demeanor and relatedness (observation of the patient's ability to engage in the interview and how they engage)	Cooperative, pleasant, calm Not in distress Appropriate to the situation	Uncooperative, hostile, agitated, avoidant, refusing to talk In distress Response is not consistent or congruent with the situation
Body movement (observation of whether the patient's behaviors are appropriate to the situation)	Calm	Fidgety or pacing, or they seem to be in slow motion In distress Unusual movements at baseline, particularly since many psychiatric medications can cause unusual movements

 CASE STUDY

Patient presents to clinic feeling unwell

| **T** 98.6°F oral | **HR** 70 bpm | **BP** 121/70 | **RR** 18 | **O2** 99% | **Pain** 0 |

Jourdan is a 33-year-old Afro-Caribbean assigned male at birth, and preferred pronouns are he/him. He presents to the clinic where you work in October in the northeast part of the United States for an appointment. You are the nurse who greets him in the waiting room and accompanies him to the examination room. Jourdan informs you that he has not been feeling well lately and is accompanied by his partner, Claudia, who also reports concerns for him not being himself.

QUESTION 6.1 (Fill in the blank)

What are the observable elements in the appearance section of the mental status assessment before the interaction starts with a patient?

1. _____

2. _____

3. _____

4. _____

Answer: 1. Hygiene and grooming; **2.** Dress; **3.** Behavior; **4.** Body movement

RATIONALE

A mental status exam commences with observation, starting outward and moving inward. The observations are the first pieces of the information puzzle to assess the external behaviors of a patient before moving inward to assess relatedness (Jarvis, 2016).

Behavior

The patient interview commences with deeper observations of the patient's presentation, starting with speech, affect, mood, eye contact, and level of consciousness (see Table 6.2).

Speech and fluency are evaluated passively throughout the assessment with observation of language skills and articulation. Tone of speech is the audible sound of speech of the patient. Rate of speech assesses the speed of words, while rhythm assesses the flow of words. Rhythm describes delays such as latency between questions and responses, or spontaneous responses with appropriate length of time between questions and answers.

TABLE 6.2 Documentation of Observed Presentation

Element	Findings Within Normal Limits	Atypical Findings
Speech (tone, rate, and rhythm)	Tone within normal limits Rate within normal limits Rhythm within normal limits	Loud, soft, child-like, rapid, slowed, slurred, or latency

continues

TABLE 6.2 Documentation of Observed Presentation *(continued)*

Element	Findings Within Normal Limits	Atypical Findings
Fluency (ability to choose appropriate vocabulary and sentence structure)	Fluent	Word-finding difficulties Note: If the patient's native language is different from the language being used during the assessment, this may contribute to difficulty with vocabulary and not indicative of altered mental status or neurocognitive disorder.
Content and coherence (ability to organize thoughts and stay on topic)	Clear, organized, and relatable	Difficult to understand or follow
Eye contact (level of consistency in looking in practitioner's eyes during the interaction, as appropriate to patient's culture)	Maintains appropriate eye contact	Minimal, avoidant, intense, poor, or no eye contact
Level of consciousness (ability to stay alert, awake, and aware while appropriately responding to stimuli such as questions and conversations)	Alert and aware Energetic or animated	Confused Sleepy, sluggish (lethargic) Apathetic (lacking interest)
Affect (emotional expression during the interview that assesses range and appropriateness to the situation)	Congruent (appropriate to situation) Full range of affect	Incongruent (not appropriate to situation) Overly excitable Flat or unchanged
Mood (subjective description of patient when asked, "How are you feeling today?"; assessed for appropriateness)	"Happy" "Worried" "Sad, depressed" "Angry"	

Patient information continued... After vital signs are taken, the nurse asks Jourdan some more questions to better understand how he has been doing. Jourdan looks down at the floor while answering and can barely be heard when he speaks. He describes his mood as "so-so," and he is aware and awake but sluggish. He describes attending the appointment today due to low energy, decreased appetite, and poor sleep. He denies any past psychiatric history or substance abuse. He recently lost a close friend, and the funeral was two weeks ago.

QUESTION 6.2 (Multiple response)

What information from the case vignette above would identify the patient's mood?

A) Jourdan is bright and engaging.

B) He is feeling "so-so."

C) Speech is described as low tone and volume.

D) Jourdan's level of consciousness is awake and aware of the situation.

Answer: B

RATIONALE

Mood is the patient's subjective report of feelings. Figure 6.1 shows the patient with a flat affect. His speech is barely audible, described as low tone and volume, and his level of consciousness shows that he is aware of where he is, the time of day, and his current need to be seen to address concerns.

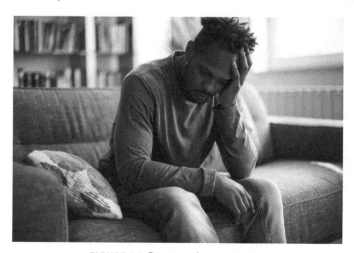

FIGURE 6.1 Depressed presentation.

QUESTION 6.3 (Fill in the blank)

Using the image in Figure 6.1 to describe appearance, fill in the blanks:

Jourdan's eye contact is _____ . His dress is _____ for the season, and his grooming is _____ .

Answer: Jourdan's eye contact is *minimal or poor*. His attire is *appropriate* for the season, and his grooming is *well-kept and clean*.

RATIONALE

Jourdan's eye contact is minimal, which could be indicative of depression despite being appropriately dressed, well-groomed, and clean. Not all elements of appearance need to be present for someone to exhibit a decline in functioning. It is important to take into account the history and timeline of the current level of functioning and changes to best understand a patient's baseline experience.

> Depending on someone's cultural background, eye contact could be viewed differently. In Eastern cultures, maintaining eye contact may be viewed as disrespectful, while in Western cultures, not maintaining eye contact may be viewed as disrespectful, aloof, or distracted. It is important to take into context the entire interaction vs. assumptions of a patient's social behaviors based on eye contact alone. Eye contact can indicate a person's feelings:
> - Short or intermittent eye contact can express nervousness, shyness, or mistrust.
> - Lack of eye contact can indicate anxiety or overt sadness.
> - Consistent eye contact can express interest or a level of comfort with the interaction.

Thought Process

Thought process assesses the way in which a patient thinks and whether the patient *makes sense*. It is the organization of thoughts that is being assessed (see Table 6.3).

TABLE 6.3 Documentation of Observed Thought Process

Element	Findings Within Normal Limits	Atypical Findings
Thought process	Logical, organized, goal-directed (clear connection between what is being said and how it is being said)	Disorganized (illogical)
		Thought blocking (long pauses)
		Circumstantial (thoughts go off on a tangent, then return to original point)
		Tangential (thoughts go off on a tangent and don't return to the original topic)

QUESTION 6.4 (Short response)

The nurse wants to clarify if there are any other areas that may be worrisome for Jourdan's reasoning and thought process. The nurse asks the following question, and Jourdan responds. Identify the type of thought process exhibited:

Nurse: "Have you noticed any changes in speed or pattern of thinking?"

Jourdan: "I sometimes feel like my thoughts are racing and I am overthinking."

How would the nurse describe Jourdan's thought process?

_____

_____

_____

Answer: Organized and logical

RATIONALE

Jourdan is aware that he has been experiencing thoughts that appear to be racing lately, consistent with overthinking. He exhibits clear, logical, and goal-directed thinking (Jarvis, 2016).

QUESTION 6.5 (Short response)

The nurse asks the following question, and Jourdan responds. Identify the type of thought process exhibited:

Nurse: "Jourdan, tell me about your morning routine."

Jourdan: "I usually wake up at 6:30 a.m. and see the sun come up. There's mail in the kitchen that I checked this morning where I left my keys yesterday. I needed to get gas, so I grabbed my keys. I saw my neighbor, and we had a quick chat about the weather while I was putting something in the mailbox. Anyway, I usually make some tea and then wake up the kids. I went to check on some tomatoes I planted but realized the squirrels kept stealing them. I eventually left to get gas and came back."

How would the nurse describe Jourdan's thought process?

_____

_____

_____

Answer: Circumstantial

RATIONALE

Jourdan's response demonstrates a *circumstantial* thought process characterized by excessive and unnecessary details. He goes off on tangents, providing additional information that may not be relevant to the question at hand about the morning routine. He eventually returns to the topic but digresses along the way (Jarvis, 2016).

Thought Content

The thought content section of the mental status exam assesses for risk and safety, as well as the subject matter of the patient's thoughts, called perceptions. Specifically assessed is impairment in perception, which is the presence of difficulty differentiating between what is reality and what might be a disturbance in reality, such as delusions, illusions, or hallucinations.

Risk and Safety

Patients may experience feelings of guilt, helplessness, or worthlessness that can contribute to the risk for physical harm to themselves or others. Many variables can contribute to this experience, such as grief and loss, new health issues, change to employment status, or change in relationship status. It is important to ask about safety and be comfortable with asking affirmative questions that are closed-ended (yes or no responses) to clarify safety concerns. It sometimes feels uncomfortable to ask about risk and safety due to your own discomfort with the information being shared by the patient. The myth is that if you ask the question, the question may spark an idea in the patient. This belief is false. Asking the question does not plant ideas in a patient's mind. It is important to note that not all patients diagnosed with depression experience suicidal ideation, and not all patients who experience suicidal ideation are diagnosed with depression. Although the experience of suicidal ideation is debilitating, its disclosure often indicates the patient's willingness to receive help. If information is disclosed in an interaction, promptly inform a mental health professional, or connect the patient with the nearest available resource for further assessment and evaluation.

Questions to elicit safety and risk are generalized to elicit the presence of thoughts of self-harm, thoughts of harm to others, and thoughts about dying, with further clarification about plan, means, and intent asked more specifically.

General assessment of presence of safety concerns:

- Do you ever experience thoughts of harming yourself or others?
- Have you ever experienced thoughts about causing your own death?

- How often do you experience these thoughts?
- Have you ever acted on these thoughts in the past?

Assessing plan:

- Have you ever created a plan?
- What is the plan?

Assessing means:

- Do you have access to follow through with the plan?
- Have you explored getting access to the means to follow through with the plan, such as researching information via the internet?

Assessing intent:

- Do you have any intention of following through with the plan?
- What has stopped you from following through with the plan?

> *Patient information continued...* Jourdan completed a PHQ-9 assessment and a GAD-7. He scored 18/27 on the PHQ-9 and 12/21 on the GAD-7. The nurse proceeds to ask clarifying questions about the responses on the assessments. Jourdan explains that he has been feeling depressed and has been suffering with "thoughts that he would be better off dead, or of hurting himself nearly every day." He reports that he has been feeling increasingly stressed about hearing God's voice.

QUESTION 6.6 (Multiple response)

The nurse needs to ask clarifying questions to Jourdan about his response on the PHQ-9 regarding safety. Identify the question that solicits the most information: *(Select all that apply)*

A) Jourdan, you have thoughts "nearly every day" about "hurting yourself or being better off dead." What stops you from acting on those thoughts?

B) Jourdan, I noticed you listed "nearly every day" for the question about "thoughts that you would be better off dead or thoughts of hurting yourself." Do you have a specific plan or intent to act on those thoughts right now or have you in the last few weeks?

C) Have you ever had thoughts of hurting yourself or acted on thoughts to cause your own death in the past?

D) Do you know why you are feeling unsafe?

Answer: A, B, and C

RATIONALE

All of the responses ask directly about the history or current presence of thoughts regarding intent or plan to assess the immediacy of the safety concern and current safety risk level except for D. The presence of a history of self-harm behaviors or previous suicide attempts increases safety risks. Response D assesses insight rather than safety risks (Jarvis, 2016).

Perceptions

Questions about perceptual experiences such as hallucinations, paranoia, or sensory distortions assess a patient's capacity to maintain awareness of reality. Perceptions are considered the *subject matter* of the patient's thoughts. A common way to elicit perceptions is through direct questions to obtain information:

Paranoia: Are you feeling watched or controlled?

Delusions (fixed beliefs not based in reality): Are you having delusions? If so, about what?

Phobias: Are you afraid of any specific things, places, or experiences?

Hallucinations (can be experienced through any of the five senses): Do you hear things that other people may not hear? Do you see things that other people may not see? Do you smell things that are not present? Do you ever feel sensations on your body without anyone or anything present to cause them? Do you ever taste something that is not being eaten?

Observe the patient's affect during their responses. Is the thought content consistent with their affect? Does the patient appear distressed or relaxed?

The following are examples of atypical answers to questions that assess perception:

1. **Question:** Do you feel like you are being watched, controlled, or followed?

   Response: I think someone is following me when I am driving.

   This is an example of concerns for paranoia that warrants further clarification.

2. **Question:** Do you ever experience situations that make you uncomfortable?

   Response: I think when people are laughing, it's because they can see the insects crawling on me.

   This is an example of paranoia, delusions, and tactile hallucinations and warrants further clarification.

3. **Question:** Do you ever experience sensations from your senses that other people don't experience?

   Response: I hear my name being called even when there's no one at home.

   This is an example of possible experiences of auditory hallucinations that warrants further clarification.

QUESTION 6.7 (Multiple response)

What areas of the mental status exam assess suicidal ideation, homicidal ideation, delusions, and paranoia? *(Select all that apply)*

A) Thought process   **C)** Thought content

B) Safety risk assessment   **D)** Concentration

Answer: B and C

RATIONALE

Suicidal ideation, homicidal ideation, delusions, and paranoia are all areas of the mental status exam that are considered when assessing safety and risk. An inability to reality test or maintain safety with absence of intent or plan to harm oneself or others, and the presence and inability to challenge delusions or paranoia, increase the likelihood of unsafe outcomes. Those variables are consistent with thought content and refer to the specific ideas, beliefs, or perceptions that dominate a person's thinking. During a mental status exam, thought content gives insight into a patient's beliefs, perceptions, and preoccupations (Jarvis, 2016).

QUESTION 6.8 (Multiple response)

Jourdan explains that he has been hearing God's voice that "change is coming." What question would you ask to clarify and better understand Jourdan's experience? *(Select all that apply)*

A) Jourdan, would you like to talk to the provider about your hallucinations?

B) Jourdan, can you help me understand what your experience of hearing God's voice means to you?

C) Jourdan, does hearing God's voice feel distressing to you?

D) I think you might need medications for hallucinations; do you want me to make a referral?

Answer: B and C

🦉 RATIONALE

It is imperative to avoid the implicit, subjective, and personal beliefs of the nurse to cloud the assessment of a patient's beliefs and perceptions. Clarification of Jourdan's experience to assess if it is causing distress or dysfunction is important in addition to understanding what role it plays.

> Consider cultural experiences of spirituality and religious beliefs uniquely to the person, what role they play, and whether the experiences are *ego syntonic*, meaning ideas that are acceptable to the self that are consistent with one's beliefs, personality, and values as well as ways of thinking. On the other hand, a distressing experience is *ego dystonic*, meaning inconsistent with beliefs. Hearing voices is not always synonymous with a psychotic experience. Some people experience their conscious thoughts or higher self as a voice through meditation or other spiritual practices; therefore, hearing voices should not be assumed to be psychosis unless other symptoms are present that contribute to distress.

Cognition

The patient interaction continues to unfold with more data collection in the assessment. *Cognition* refers to a patient's mental processes relating to gathering and understanding information. The elements of assessment in the cognition section of the mental status exam involve memory, problem-solving, logic, reasoning, and attention.

Memory

Memory is discretely assessed via recent (short-term) memory and remote (long-term) memory.

An example of a way to elicit short-term memory is to give three items of different categories at a certain point during the interview and allow the interview to progress for five to seven minutes, then ask for the patient to recall the items asked previously. Example: book, flower, and train; or numbers such as 2, 195, and 78.

For younger children, a consideration for assessing recent memory might be the name of their teacher, and for remote memory, what date is their birthday. Ensure the questions are appropriate for the child's age and development for accuracy.

For the older population, a consideration for assessing recent memory might include asking their current address and the names of their children and grandchildren. An inability to recall may be cause for concerns relating to a decline in memory due to other reasons than aging. An example of eliciting long-term memory is to ask the patient the address where they lived in youth or the date of an important event in their life.

Patient information continued... Jourdan is aware of where he is, the general time of day, and the day of the week, and he was able to follow directions completely. The nurse asks him to recall the following four items to assess memory: loyalty, carrot, ankle, tulip. Jourdan was able to recall the words "carrot" and "ankle," but only after five minutes. However, he recalls his birthday and the birthdays of his two children.

QUESTION 6.9 (Check the correct column)

In Table 6.4, identify which questions are recent or remote memory questions:

TABLE 6.4 Recent or Remote Memory Questions

Event	Recent Memory	Remote Memory
What day of the week is it, and what time is it?		
What did you eat for breakfast?		
When are your children's birthdays?		
What time is your appointment today?		
What medications did you take today?		
What year did you migrate to the US?		

Answer Key to Question 6.9

Event	Recent Memory	Remote Memory
What day of the week is it, and what time is it?	X	
What did you eat for breakfast?	X	
When are your children's birthdays?		X
What time is your appointment today?	X	
What medications did you take today?	X	
What year did you migrate to the US?		X

RATIONALE

Recent memories are also considered short-term memories that manage the information required to carry out tasks such as learning, reasoning, and comprehension. Remote memories are also considered long-term memories or autobiographical information stored in a different part of the brain.

Logic, Reasoning, and Attention

This is the section of the mental status exam where attention is assessed. The use of simple mathematical problems or spelling can ascertain important information. Methods of collecting data include asking a patient to count by sevens or spell the word "world" backwards. Awareness of person, place, time, and situation assesses for orientation. General information can also be requested on current affairs to assess the patient's knowledge base. Additionally, questions about how to resolve an issue can be utilized to assess problem-solving capacity. Be sure to ask questions unique to the patient's lifestyle, such as asking a social media manager how to post content in order of steps to assess the patient based on experience and interest. Visual and spatial ability can be assessed by asking the patient to draw a face on a clock and set the hands to a particular time.

QUESTION 6.10 (Short responses)

Sometimes it is helpful to assess cognitive thinking by asking open-ended questions. Identify a question for each of the following to assess 1) logic and reasoning, 2) problem-solving, and 3) attention.

Fill in the blanks with three questions (Jarvis, 2016):

1. _____

2. _____

3. _____

Possible answers:

1. **Logic and reasoning question:** What would you do if you found a wallet?
2. **Problem-solving question:** How would you handle a situation where you feel overwhelmed or stressed?
3. **Attention question:** Ask the patient to spell "world" backwards.

RATIONALE
The answers above are possible responses.

Questions should elicit information to assess the patient's abilities relating to logic and reasoning, explore basic knowledge and capacity to use critical thinking, and assess the patient's morals and beliefs.

Atypical Responses to Cognitive Questions
Logic and Reasoning
Following are some examples of abnormal responses to a question that assesses logic and reasoning:

1. **Question:** What is the meaning of the following statement: "If you live in a glass house, don't throw stones."

   Response: The glass is bulletproof, and nothing will happen.

   Rationale: This response is concerning, as most windows are not bulletproof in someone's home where they live, and stones and bullets are not the same. Additionally, the statement is metaphorical, which suggests that you should not be critical of someone or a situation when you may be exhibiting the same behaviors.

2. **Question:** What is the name of the continent that the US is part of?

   Response: The US is the continent.

   Rationale: Fund of knowledge is poor, as North America consists of 23 countries including the US, which is one of the largest.

3. **Question:** If you found a cellphone, what would you do?

   Response: I would sell it.

   Rationale: This response questions if the patient is morally sound. If something of value is found that belongs to someone else, keeping it and using it for your own benefit vs. exploring mechanisms for returning it to the owner questions the patient's moral capacity to make good decisions.

Problem-Solving and Attention Span
Problem-solving and attention span questions assess the patient's capacity to think about the most appropriate way to manage a situation and the ability to stay present and focused for the assessment.

Following are some examples of abnormal responses to a question that assesses problem-solving and attention span:

1. **Question:** It's 10 a.m. Lisa and James are traveling to the airport from different locations. Lisa lives 20 minutes away, and James lives 45 minutes away. What time would each of them need to leave to get to the airport one hour before their flight at 3 p.m.?

   Response: They would leave at the same time.

   Rationale: This response is not exercising the use of critical thinking with regard to difference in distance warranting more time for the commute to arrive at the same time.

2. **Question:** You have three assignments due this week, with a makeup work assignment because you haven't been doing well academically. You are scheduled to work three 8-hour shifts this week, and a party you really want to attend is out of town. How do you prioritize based on rank of importance?

   Response: I would turn in the assignments late and take the deduction in grade for the assignments because I really don't want to miss the party, and I can't miss work because bills need to be paid.

   Rationale: The work shifts provide income for basic needs and quality of life, which are a priority. Submitting academic assignments on time contributes to grades being scored without the risk for deductions due to late submission, with the added caveat that there are academic concerns already identified, and the assignments are for opportunities to improve the grades. Choosing to attend a party out of town is not prioritizing the current needs.

3. **Question:** Ask the patient to recall items such as carrot, book, and pen, and then ask the patient to repeat the words at a later time in the assessment to assess capacity to remember and pay attention.

   Rationale: If the patient can only recall one or two items, they may be struggling with attentional difficulties or have a neurological concern that impacts memory. Note that recall of items to assess recent memory can simultaneously assess attention, since memory and attention are closely correlated.

Insight and Judgment

Insight is an internalized process and is defined as a patient's understanding of their impairment and ability to function. Documentation of insight is usually described as limited, poor, or fair and—if there is previous comparison available—worsening versus improving.

Judgment is an externalized behavior and defined as a patient's ability to understand and make good decisions. Judgment is assessed by asking a patient what they would do in specific scenarios. Like insight, judgment is also rated as poor, limited, fair, or—if there is a previous evaluation to compare to—worsening versus improving. (See Table 6.5.)

TABLE 6.5 Documentation of Insight and Judgment

Element	Findings Within Normal Limits	Atypical Findings
Insight (internal understanding of one's impairment or ability to function)	Fair, good, or improving	Limited, poor, or worsening
Judgment (ability to understand and make good decisions)	Fair, good, or improving	Limited, poor, or worsening

QUESTION 6.11 (Fill in the blanks)

The nurse asks the following questions. For each question, indicate what is being assessed.

A) Can you tell me how you perceive your current situation or the difficulties you are experiencing?

_____

B) If you were faced with a similar situation in the future, how would you handle it?

_____

C) What steps are you taking to address the current concerns that are affecting your daily functioning?

_____

D) Do you think your thoughts or behaviors might be influenced by a mental health decline?

_____

Answer: a. Insight; **b.** Judgment; **c.** Judgment; **d.** Insight

RATIONALE

A. **Insight:** This question is assessing Jourdan's self-awareness and understanding of the current difficulties creating an impairment in functioning.

B. **Judgment:** This question assesses decision-making capacity and how Jourdan would respond in the future if faced with a specific situation.

C. **Judgment:** This question assesses next steps and reasoning ability to determine next steps.

D. **Insight:** This question assesses self-awareness and is an example of an internalized process to gather information on the patient's understanding of impairment and functioning.

REFERENCE

Jarvis, C. (2016). *Physical examination and health assessment* (7th ed.). Saunders.

CHAPTER 7

Assessment Considerations for the Geriatric Patient

Louis E. D'Onofrio Jr., DNP, MSN, FNP-C, PCCN
Kristi Maynard, EdD, APRN, FNP-BC, CNE

 CASE STUDY

Geriatric Patient Presenting With Confusion

- 72-year-old male
- Presenting to the PCP with intermittent confusion

| **T** 97.0°F oral | **HR** 92 bpm | **RR** 14 | **BP** 128/70 | **O2** 97% | **Pain** 1/10 |

Mr. Hanks, a 72-year-old male, presents to the primary care outpatient office accompanied by his son. The patient is intermittently confused. The patient's son reports that they live together, and he has noticed his father's memory has worsened over the past two months. The son reports that his father has not had a primary care visit in the last four years and has never seen a gerontologist. Mr. Hanks's son is worried that something was missed over the years his father was neglecting care; he would like to start "from scratch" and also address his "memory problems."

QUESTION 7.1 (Multiple choice)

Gerontology is the study of:

A) Only the diseases unique to the aging population

B) The elderly population with mental health issues

C) The aging person and their social, cognitive, biological, and psychological aspects

D) Adult diseases

Answer: C

RATIONALE

Gerontology is the study of older adults and aging by means of a multi-disciplinary approach. Gerontology focuses on the aging person and includes cognitive, biological, social, and psychological topics of those aging. *Geriatrics* is a specific medical specialty focused on the care and treatment of older adults. A *geriatrician* is a medical provider that specializes in the aging population and the medical conditions associated with aging.

The projected number of US residents aged 65 and older by the year 2060 is 95 million (Population Reference Bureau, 2019). With an increase in our aging population, it is crucial to think about medical risk factors associated with aging. As we all age, it is normal for every organ system to undergo changes. Visual acuity decreases, cerumen production and hearing loss increase, muscle mass and strength decline, and the immune system undergoes changes that make it difficult to fight infection (Jaul & Barron, 2017). One of the most common chronic diseases in older adults is hypertension, and cancer is the second cause of death in older adults (Jaul & Barron, 2017). With many changes occurring during aging, it is important for nurses to have strong assessment skills to identify problems early and respond to this steadily growing population.

QUESTION 7.2 (Multiple response)

Which of the following subjective information collected during the health history would be considered a risk factor for dementia? *(Select all that apply)*

A) Hypertension

B) Being above age 65

C) Having type 2 diabetes

D) Alcohol usage

E) Owning a dog

F) Latex allergy

Answer: A, B, C, D

RATIONALE

Dementia is a general term used to describe a decline in memory, language, or other thinking skills. According to the Alzheimer's Society, the biggest risk factor for dementia is aging (Llewellyn, 2021). Alzheimer's disease or vascular dementia risks double every five years above the age of 65 (Llewellyn, 2021, p. 5). Medical conditions such as obesity, elevated cholesterol, hypertension, type 2 diabetes, depression, smoking, low physical exercise, and excessive alcohol use all may also increase the risk for dementia (Llewellyn, 2021). Genetics may also play a role in a person's risk for dementia.

Acute confusion or memory impairments can be the result of a lack of vitamin B1 (thiamine), and this disorder is called *Wernicke's encephalopathy*. It has been related to people with alcohol use disorders, as poor eating habits or frequent vomiting reduce B1 levels eaten or absorbed. Alcohol can also inflame the stomach lining, which may interfere with vitamin absorption (Alzheimer Scotland, 2004). People with eating disorders, renal problems, GI absorption conditions, or severe vomiting can also experience vitamin B1 deficiencies.

Alcohol screening is always a good idea to try to identify those with possible alcohol use disorders. Traditionally the four-question tool (known as the *CAGE questionnaire*) has played an important role in the identification of alcohol dependency. These questions are:

1. Have you ever desired to cut down on your drinking?
2. Have you ever felt annoyance when your drinking has been criticized?
3. Have you ever felt guilty about your drinking?
4. Have you ever experienced an eye-opening moment?

The helpful and well-known mnemonic "CAGE" stands for: Cut down, Annoyed, Guilty, and Eye-opener. Two positive questions on a CAGE questionnaire was considered positive, but now even one positive answer should trigger further investigation to rule out substance abuse (Ewing, 1984).

QUESTION 7.3 (Multiple choice)

When evaluating the geriatric patient, the nurse is *incorrect* in stating:

A) Aging includes many physiological changes.

B) There are special considerations for mental health in the geriatric patient.

C) There are no specific changes associated with aging.

D) Safety is a major issue in geriatric patients with declining functional status.

Answer: C

RATIONALE

As a person ages, there are many "normal" variants of aging. You may recognize some of the more obvious changes with simple inspection. An example may be the hair turning gray or white as melanin production decreases, or the skin beginning to wrinkle or sag with loss of elasticity. While this presentation may not appear "normal" compared to the examination of a healthy young adult, these are normal variants of aging.

QUESTION 7.4 (Fill in the blank)

The nurse recognizes that the geriatric patient may experience physiological and psychological changes associated with aging. List three potential changes considered to be normal variants of aging.

1. _____

2. _____

3. _____

ANSWER(S)/RATIONALE

There are many changes associated with aging; some include (Mayo Clinic, 2023):

- Decreased bone density
- Loss of muscle strength and flexibility
- Increased likelihood of constipation
- Decreased bladder control or increased frequency of urination
- Decreased memory or ability to multitask
- Loss of close vision
- Development of cataracts
- High-frequency hearing loss
- Dry mouth
- Gum disease
- Thinning of the skin, loss of elasticity causing wrinkles, and age spots
- Decreased metabolism

QUESTION 7.5 (Multiple response)

When assessing the elder adult, the nurse recognizes which blood pressure to be in normal range for a patient > 65 years old? (Select all that apply)

A) 128/78

B) 134/80

C) 120/90

D) 90/56

Answer: D

RATIONALE

Starting in 2017, the American Heart Association and the American College of Cardiology were among some of the many organizations that adjusted the blood pressure ranges used to diagnosis hypertension. The previous American Heart Association guidelines had set thresholds at 140/90 mmHg for those younger than 65 and 150/80mmHg for those 65 or older. Now clinical judgment is advised for those older than 65 years old by the American College of Cardiology, and most new blood pressure guidelines support lower than 120/80mmHg as the nonhypertensive range and anything over that to be elevated or hypertensive (Whelton et al., 2018).

QUESTION 7.6 (Multiple response)

In this chapter's case scenario, Mr. Hanks has not seen a provider for health screenings in several years. Mr. Hanks most likely missed some routine health screenings that are age-appropriate. Which of the below are age-appropriate screenings for patients age 65 or older? *(Select all that apply)*

A) Abdominal aortic aneurysm (AAA)

B) Lung cancer chest CT

C) Bone density/DEXA scan

D) Dix-Hallpike

E) Electrocardiogram (ECG)

F) Prostate-specific antigen (PSA)

G) Mammogram

H) Colonoscopy

I) Checking for a Murphy's sign

Answer: A, B, C, F, G, H

RATIONALE

The US Preventive Services Task Force is an independent panel of experts that review evidence and develop recommendations for preventive services (2019). Based on the US Preventive Services Task Force, guidelines may change based on updated research. The following data were reviewed in December 2019. For the most up-to-date guidelines, visit https://www.uspreventiveservicestaskforce.org/.

Patient information continued... Mr. Hanks and his son have agreed to take part in age-appropriate screenings and have discussed risk factors associated with dementia. The patient reported he did smoke cigarettes—about half a pack per day for 10 years in his thirties, then stopped in his forties—and denies hypertension or diabetes issues known. Mr. Hanks completed the provider-driven SLUMS testing and scored an 18. Mr. Hanks reports he did not graduate college but did finish high school. Mr. Hanks asked the nurse what other things can cause acute memory loss and would like to know more about the SLUMS test and what the score means.

QUESTION 7.7 (Multiple choice)

What is a SLUMS test?

A) Another name for a Mini-Mental State Exam

B) An examination to detect mild cognitive impairments and dementia

C) An exam to determine if a patient is in financial trouble or at risk for being homeless

D) An assessment for elder violence

Answer: B

RATIONALE

The SLUMS test is short for the Saint Louis University Mental Status examination and is used for screening and detecting dementia or cognitive impairments. The SLUMS has also been considered a more accurate tool for screening for cognitive impairments by some studies (Szczesniak & Rymaszewska, 2016). The SLUMS examination allows the provider to ask questions, for which each question has a point value. At the end of the exam, the points are totaled. The scoring ranges are different for patients who completed high school and those who have not. The ranges are at the bottom of the test form and can be observed in Table 7.1.

TABLE 7.1 SLUMS Scoring Ranges

SLUMS Scoring		
High School Education		**Less Than High School Education**
27–30	Normal	20–30
20–27	MCI	14–19
1–19	Dementia	1–14

(Szczesniak & Rymaszewska, 2016)

Many other medical conditions can cause memory issues. Syphilis, Lyme disease, and urinary tract infections are a few infections known to cause memory or cognition issues. Active infections should always be ruled out for new reported patient concerns related to their memory because these may cause a SLUMS score to be abnormal. Vitamin deficiencies may also be a cause of memory issues, such as B12 or previously mentioned B1.

Medications can be helpful for many patients, but all medications have side effect risks. An issue of concern for the aging population is always medication errors and *polypharmacy* (taking a large amount of medications). Some medications, such as antibiotics, have been known to cause encephalopathy (Bhattacharyya et al., 2016). When the brain is being affected by an agent, such as an antibiotic, or condition, such as a virus, a patient can have memory and cognitive impairments.

When a person has a cerebrovascular accident (CVA), more commonly known as a stroke, memory loss often occurs. During a CVA, nerve cells in the brain become damaged and lost. How a person's memory suffers all depends on the location of the CVA; for instance, verbal memory or visual memory all depend on which side of the brain was damaged (Novitzke, 2008).

Patient information continued... Mr. Hanks completed all his laboratory tests and had no indication of having an infection, vitamin deficiency, or medication that has caused his recent memory concerns. Mr. Hanks and his son reported that Mr. Hanks fell and hit his head recently and was seen in a local emergency department. When the nurse reviews recent imaging, it appears his head CT was normal, and no CVA was reported. Mr. Hanks is due to establish care with a geriatric specialist for his suspected dementia, and his son has concerns about him falling at home.

QUESTION 7.8 (Multiple response)

What are risk factors for a patient falling in the home? *(Select all that apply)*

A) Fear of falling

B) Impaired walking

C) Dim lighting at home

D) Living alone

E) Poor reaction time

Answer: A, B, C, E

RATIONALE

There are many risk factors associated with falls. Some intrinsic factors include advanced age, fall history, weakness, visual loss, fear of falling, and some chronic diseases (Parkinson's, dementia, arthritis, stroke). Extrinsic factors, which can be modified, are lack of working stair handrails, poor stair design, lack of bathroom grab bars, dim lighting, tripping hazards, slippery surfaces, psychoactive medications, and improperly used assistive devices. To help prevent a patient from falling, the patient, patient's family, and provider must create and meet goals. Some interventions to reduce fall risks may include reviewing medication for safety, balance training, learning how to use walking devices properly, and strength training.

Patient information continued... Mr. Hanks has been on a cognition-enhancing medication and has had stable SLUMS scores. He has been taking part in local community center fall prevention exercise classes and denies any new falls. Mr. Hanks's son reports following a home safety plan that the geriatric provider advised. Mr. Hanks now has a laminated medication list and emergency numbers in his wallet, safety grab bars in the shower, nonslip pads in the shower, and newly installed smoke detectors, and the home is free of floor clutter. Mr. Hanks's son would like you, his nurse, to suggest other safety tips that can be done in the home to prevent falls.

QUESTION 7.9 (Fill in the blank)

Mr. Hanks's son is interested in making some modifications around the house to reduce the risk of falls for his elderly father. What are three potential home modifications that may help reduce falls?

1. _____

2. _____

3. _____

ANSWER(S)/RATIONALE

Simple home modifications may help improve the safety of the elderly patient in their home environment. Some changes the nurse may recommend include removing any clutter from the floor, arranging furniture to allow for adequate walking space, placing nonslip pads on steps and under rugs, salting driveways and steps during icy weather, ensuring adequate lighting, and properly installing handrails and guardrails, especially in challenging areas like the bathtub (National Council on Aging, 2023). According to Phelan et al. (2015), fall risk in the elderly is a combination of individual (intrinsic) and environmental (extrinsic) factors. Physiological changes that may increase the risk of falls are highlighted in Table 7.2.

TABLE 7.2 Intrinsic Changes Impacting Fall Risk

Organ System	Physiological Change	
Muscular system	Decreased muscle strength	
Nervous system	Balance	Increased postural sway
		Slow reflexes
	Gait	Decreased step height
		Decreased proprioception
	Vision	Reduced pupillary response to light variation
		Thickening of lenses

(Phelan et al., 2015)

QUESTION 7.10 (Multiple choice)

When performing a formal fall-risk assessment, the nurse recognizes the most accurate way to evaluate fall risk is by:

A) Observing the patient for high-risk behavior

B) Asking family members their opinion on the patient's safety

C) Performing a comprehensive in-home assessment

D) Utilizing a combination of evidence-based screening tools

Answer: D

RATIONALE

The most effective method of evaluating fall risk is using a combination of evidence-based fall assessment tools. While use of a single assessment tool may be predictive, Park (2018) found that using a combination of tools was more predictive and accurate than use of any tool alone.

Patient information continued... Mr. Hanks has been managing his care at home with the assistance of his son. One morning, Mr. Hanks slipped and fell on an icy sidewalk while attempting to retrieve the morning paper. An ORIF was performed, and the patient was admitted to a short-term rehabilitation to regain strength before returning home. After four weeks, it has been determined that Mr. Hanks may return home with visiting nursing services and home physical therapy visits. He will follow up with his primary care provider and orthopedist on a regular basis.

QUESTION 7.11 (Multiple choice)

A critical function of the nurse is medication reconciliation. The process of medication reconciliation is *best* described as:

A) Counting all pills before the patient is discharged from hospital to home

B) Educating the patient and family on medication side effects

C) Cross-checking documentation of prescribed medications for redundancies, errors, or safety concerns as a patient transfers from one environment to another

D) Purchasing over-the-counter medications to supplement prescription medications

Answer: C

RATIONALE

Medication reconciliation is an important process to minimize medication errors as a patient is transitioned from one facility to another. This may be from the hospital to a short-term rehabilitation center or even to the patient's home. As many as one in six patients will have a medication discrepancy occur upon transfer. A thorough reconciliation can reduce the nearly 30% likelihood of a patient incurring harm as a result of a medication error (Duguid, 2012). Elderly patients may be at an increased risk for medication errors, especially if they suffer from conditions like Alzheimer's or dementia that impair their cognitive abilities.

QUESTION 7.12 (Multiple choice)

The visiting nurse is making her first visit to Mr. Hanks this morning. During her visit, she notes a new prescription from the orthopedist for a pain medication and a second new prescription from his primary care provider for a sleeping aid. In total, Mr. Hanks is prescribed eight medications. The nurse recognizes this medication combination is potentially serious and alerts the prescribers. What term best describes this situation?

A) Polypharmacy

B) Drug addiction

C) Pill hoarding

D) Prior authorization

Answer: A

RATIONALE

Polypharmacy is described as an individual with five or more prescribed daily medications (Masnoon et al., 2017). The likelihood of polypharmacy increases in individuals with multiple medical conditions requiring prescription management. The risk can be exacerbated if specialists and caregivers are not maintaining contact regarding their medical plan of care or recommended prescriptions. Since the elderly are more likely to be diagnosed with multiple comorbidities, they are at an increased risk for polypharmacy (Masnoon et al., 2017). Polypharmacy can become dangerous when medications interact or side effects of one medication compound another.

CHAPTER 7 WORKSHEET

Based on my initial assessment, I thought:

_____

_____

_____

Based on my revised/informed assessment, I now know:

_____

_____

_____

A nursing priority for this patient would be _____

because _____

After completing this chapter, something I have learned is:

_____

_____

_____

After completing this chapter, something I need more clarity on is:

_____

_____

_____

After completing this chapter, something else I want to learn is:

_____

_____

_____

REFERENCES

Alzheimer Scotland. (2004). Alcohol-related brain damage—Wernicke's encephalopathy and Korsakoff's psychosis. *Information Sheet, 31*, 1–4. https://www.alzscot.org/sites/default/files/images/0000/0166/alcohol.pdf

Bhattacharyya, S., Darby, R. R., Raibagkar, P., Gonzalez Castro, L. N., & Berkowitz, A. L. (2016). Antibiotic-associated encephalopathy. *Neurology, 86*(10), 963–971. https://doi.org/10.1212/WNL.0000000000002455

Duguid, M. (2012). The importance of medication reconciliation for patients and practitioners. *Australian Prescriber, 35*(1), 15–19. https://doi.org/10.18773/austprescr.2012.007

Ewing, J. A. (1984). Detecting alcoholism: The CAGE questionnaire. *JAMA, 252*(14), 1905–1907. https://doi.org/10.1001/jama.1984.03350140051025

National Council on Aging. (2023). *Home modification tools and tips to help prevent falls.* https://www.ncoa.org/article/home-modification-tools-and-tips-to-help-prevent-falls

Jaul, E., & Barron, J. (2017). Age-related diseases and clinical and public health implications for the 85 years old and over population. *Frontiers in Public Health, 5*, 335. https://doi.org/10.3389/fpubh.2017.00335

Llewellyn, D. (2021). *Risk factors for dementia.* Alzheimer's Society. https://www.alzheimers.org.uk/sites/default/files/pdf/factsheet_risk_factors_for_dementia.pdf

Masnoon, N., Shakib, S., Kalisch-Ellett, L., & Caughey, G. E. (2017). What is polypharmacy? A systematic review of definitions. *BMC Geriatrics, 17*, 230. https://doi.org/10.1186/s12877-017-0621-2

Mayo Clinic. (2023, September 20). *Aging: What to expect.* https://www.mayoclinic.org/healthy-lifestyle/healthy-aging/in-depth/aging/art-20046070

Novitzke, J. (2008). Privation of memory: What can be done to help stroke patients remember? *Journal of Vascular and Interventional Neurology, 1*(4), 122–123.

Park, S. H. (2018). Tools for assessing fall risk in the elderly: A systematic review and meta-analysis. *Aging Clinical and Experimental Research, 30*(1), 1–16. https://doi.org/10.1007/s40520-017-0749-0

Phelan, E. A., Mahoney, J. E., Voit, J. C., & Stevens, J. A. (2015). Assessment and management of fall risk in primary care settings. *Medical Clinics, 99*(2), 281–293. https://doi.org/10.1016/j.mcna.2014.11.004

Population Reference Bureau. (2019). *Fact sheet: Aging in the United States.* https://www.prb.org/aging-unitedstates-fact-sheet/

Szczesniak, D., & Rymaszewska, J. (2016). The usefulness of the SLUMS test for diagnosis of mild cognitive impairment and dementia. *Polish Psychiatry, 50*(2), 457–72. https://doi.org/10.12740/PP/OnlineFirst/43141

US Preventive Services Task Force. (2019). *About the USPSTF.* https://www.uspreventiveservicestaskforce.org/uspstf/about-uspstf

Whelton, P., Carey, R., Aronow, W., Casey, D., Collins, K., Dennison Himmelfarb, C., DePalma, S., Gidding, S., Jamerson, K., Jones, D., MacLaughlin, E., Muntner, P., Ovbiagele, B., Smith, S. C., Spencer, C. C., Stafford, R., Taler, S., Thomas, R., Williams, K., Williamson, J., & Wright, J. (2018). 2017 ACC/AHA/AAPA/ABC/ACPM/ AGS/APhA/ASH/ASPC/NMA/PCNA guideline for the prevention, detection, evaluation, and management of high blood pressure in adults: A report of the American College of Cardiology/American Heart Association Task Force on Clinical Practice Guidelines. *Hypertension, 71*(6), 1269–1324. https://www.ahajournals.org/doi/epub/10.1161/HYP.0000000000000065

Assessment Considerations for the Pediatric Patient

Antoinette Towle, EdD, MSN, APRN, SNP-BC, PNP-BC

 CASE STUDY

Pediatric Patient Presenting for Physical Exam

- 6-year-old female with unremarkable health history
- Grandmother present (provider of childcare while parents work)

T 98.1°F oral	**HR** 80 bpm	**RR** 24	**BP** 100/60	**O2** 99%	**Pain** 0/10

Susie Lynn, a 6-year-old female, comes to the clinic for her prekindergarten school physical examination. She is with her grandmother, Mary. Susie Lynn tells the nurse that she is so excited to be starting school in the fall with her older brother, Bobby, who will be in second grade. Mary states that she watches both Susie Lynn and Bobby every day after school and during the summer while their parents work. She has been the primary babysitter since they were both born. Mary states that Susie Lynn has been relatively healthy over the past year, having had only one cold a few months ago.

The following information was noted from the electronic health record (EHR) from her last well child visit one year ago:

Name: Susie Lynn White

Date of Birth: May 10, 2017

Age: 6

Gender: female

Ethnicity: white

Address: 123 Brown Street, Waterbury, CT 06521

Phone: (555) 274-1212

Parent(s)/Guardian: John and Kim White (parents), Mary Stone, grandmother

Language Spoken: English

Religion: Catholic

Past Medical History: repeated streptococcal pharyngitis (6/1/2018, 9/21/2018, 12/25/2018, 2/17/2019, 5/11/2019, 7/4/2019, 11/21/2019, 3/2/2020, 7/2/2020), referred ENT Specialist Dr. Nose on 2/17/2019

Past Surgical History: tonsillectomy and adenoidectomy (8/1/2020, age 3)

Family History: mother (gestational diabetes), maternal grandmother (hypertension), paternal grandfather (lung cancer)

Allergies: NKDA, NKFA

QUESTION 8.1 (Multiple choice)

The identifying data or identifiers are one component of a comprehensive pediatric health history. Which of the following is included as part of the patient's identifying data?

A) The reason for seeking care

B) Details about the history of the present illness or complaint

C) The child's past medical history

D) The child's age

Answer: D

RATIONALE

In the pediatric history, the identifying data include biographical information such as age, ethnicity, gender, occupation (i.e., student), address/phone number, and language spoken. The Joint Commission now requires documentation of patient/family language communication needs to promote patient-centered communication standards (Jarvis, 2016; The Joint Commission, 2010).

QUESTION 8.2 (Multiple response)

The components of the comprehensive pediatric health history include: *(Select all that apply)*

A) Identifying/biographic data

B) Chief complaint and history of the present illness

C) Past medical and surgical history

D) Family medical history

Answer: A, B, C, D

RATIONALE

The components of the comprehensive pediatric health history include: identifying/biographic data, chief complaint, history of the present illness, past medical history, family medical history, personal and social history, and the review of systems (Hockenberry & Wilson, 2017; Jarvis, 2016). Information obtained in a comprehensive health history is usually completed at the initial office visit and then updated at each subsequent visit as needed.

The past medical history (PMH) is a more detailed description of the child's prior health problems. When collecting information for the PMH, document (Ball et al., 2017; Bickley, 2017):

- The child's age at the time of each major illness or injury
- History of common communicable diseases (such as streptococcal pharyngitis)
- Surgical history (including one-day or outpatient surgeries)
- History of hospitalizations (along with age and dates of each event)
- History of childhood illnesses, such as recurrent ear infections or upper respiratory infections
- History of visits to any medical specialists (e.g., ear, nose, and throat; cardiology; psychiatry), medication allergies (with specific reactions, such as hives or periorbital swelling)
- Environmental and food allergies (with reactions)
- Immunizations
- Any chronic illnesses (such as asthma or diabetes)

For children 2 and under and when the child's present problem may be related to birth (e.g., cerebral palsy), the child's birth history should be included. The birth history should include information on the mother and infant.

Table 8.1 outlines what information should be included in a thorough birth history.

TABLE 8.1 Birth History

Birth History Assessment Questions	
Mother	**Infant**
Age	Place of delivery
Health during pregnancy	Vaginal or cesarean birth (reason for cesarean included)
Weight gain during pregnancy	
Initiation and length of prenatal care	Gestational age at birth
Prior obstetric history	Birth weight
History of infection and injury	Apgar score
Use of substances during pregnancy (alcohol, cigarettes, prescription drugs, marijuana, cocaine, heroin)	Postnatal course including length of hospital stay and admission to special nursery (include postnatal infection and need for antibiotics)
Complications during delivery or immediately postpartum	

(Ball et al., 2017)

Patient information continued... In reviewing Susie Lynn's EHR, her last physical examination was at age 5, dated 5/12/22. At that visit she received no immunizations. The following current immunization record was noted:

Vaccine	Date Given	Vaccine	Date Given	Vaccine	Date Given	Vaccine	Date Given
Hep B #1	5/11/17	DTaP #1	7/6/17	PCV13 #1	7/6/17	Hep A #1	5/11/18
Hep B #2	6/11/17	DTaP #2	9/2/17	PCV13 #2	9/2/17	Hep A #2	6/11/18
Hep B #3	11/14/17	DTaP #3	11/6/17	PCV13 #3	11/6/17	Varicella #1	8/4/18
RV #1	7/6/17	DTaP #4	8/4/18	PCV13 #4	5/10/18	Varicella #2	
RV #2	9/2/17	DTaP #5		IPV #1	7/6/17	Men. B #1	
RV #3	11/6/17	Hib #1	7/6/17	IPV #2	8/5/17	Men. B #2	
MMR #1	5/10/18	Hib #2	9/2/17	IPV #3	5/11/18	HPV #1	
MMR #2	5/12/21	Hib #3	11/6/17	IPV #4		HPV #2	
Tdap > 11; q 10 yrs		Hib #4	5/10/18	Influenza (yearly)* 10/1/17, 10/2/18, 10/10/19, 10/16/20, 9/30/21, 11/1/22		Meningococcal #1 (MenACWY-D)	
PPD (if required)						Meningococcal #2 (MenACWY-D)	

QUESTION 8.3 (Multiple choice)

In reviewing Susie Lynn's current immunization schedule, what immunizations will she receive on her scheduled 6-year-old well child visit?

A) DTaP #5, Varicella, IPV #4, PPD (if required)

B) DTaP #5, Varicella, IPV #4, Influenza (yearly)

C) DTaP #5, Varicella, IPV #4, Influenza (yearly), HPV #1

D) No immunizations are needed.

Answer: A

RATIONALE

The Centers for Disease Control and Prevention (CDC) annually publishes a recommended immunization schedule for children (ages 0–18 years) to reflect changes in vaccine formulations and current recommendations for the use of licensed vaccines (CDC, 2023). These schedules are available online at https://www.cdc.gov/vaccines/schedules/downloads/child/0-18yrs-child-combined-schedule.pdf. A catch-up schedule is also published by the CDC for children who have missed immunization.

QUESTION 8.4 (Multiple choice)

When should Susie Lynn receive her yearly influenza vaccine?

A) At her 6-year-old well child visit 5/10/23

B) Anytime; time does not matter with this vaccine.

C) Influenza vaccine is not needed in healthy children.

D) Preferable during the fall months, September and October

Answer: A

RATIONALE

Recommendations from the CDC regarding the influenza vaccine include (CDC, 2021):

- The influenza vaccine should be given at 6 months of age and yearly thereafter prior to flu season, usually around the month of October.
- Anyone 6 months of age and older should get vaccinated every flu season.
- Children 6 months through 8 years of age may need two doses during a single flu season. Everyone else needs only one dose each flu season.
- It takes about two weeks for protection to develop after vaccination.
- There are many flu viruses, and they are always changing.
- Each year a new flu vaccine is made to protect against three or four viruses that are likely to cause disease in the upcoming flu season.
- Even when the vaccine doesn't exactly match these viruses, it may still provide some protection.
- Influenza vaccine does not cause flu.
- Influenza vaccine may be given at the same time as other vaccines.

QUESTION 8.5 (Multiple choice)

At what age should Susie Lynn be vaccinated with the human papillomavirus (HPV) vaccine? Should she wait until she is sexually active prior to getting the vaccine?

A) Not needed if she is not sexually active

B) Two doses of HPV vaccine for all adolescents at age 11 or 12 years, prior to sexual activity

C) It can be taken at any time during adolescence, and only one dose is required.

D) The only time the HPV vaccine may be given is prior to the age of 11 and prior to sexual activity.

Answer: B

RATIONALE

According to the CDC, approximately 80% of people will get an HPV infection in their lifetime. HPV vaccination provides the most benefit when given before a person is exposed to any HPV. The CDC recommends two doses of HPV vaccine for all adolescents at age 11 or 12 years. For the HPV vaccination, a two-dose schedule is recommended for people who get the first dose before their 15th birthday. In a two-dose series, the second dose should be given six to 12 months after the first dose (0, six-to-12-month schedule). The minimum interval is five months between the first and second dose. If the second dose is administered after a shorter interval, a third dose should be administered a minimum of five months after the first dose and a minimum of 12 weeks after the second dose (CDC, 2019).

Most sexually active adults have already been exposed to HPV, although not necessarily all the HPV types targeted by vaccination. At any age, having a new sex partner is a risk factor for getting a new HPV infection. Therefore, sexually active individuals should consult with their medical provider as to the benefits of obtaining the vaccine once sexually active.

QUESTION 8.6 (Multiple choice)

The review of systems (ROS) provides a comprehensive overview of a child's health. Which of the following statements regarding the ROS is not true?

A) Identifies signs and symptoms that may be associated with the patient's condition

B) Documents the presence and absence of common symptoms related to each major body system

C) Primarily focused on disease history

D) Proceeds in a "head-to-toe" fashion

Answer: C

RATIONALE

The ROS is an additional opportunity to identify signs and symptoms that may be associated with the patient's condition (Ball et al., 2017; Jarvis, 2016). The ROS documents the presence and absence of common symptoms related to each major body system, proceeding in a "head-to-toe" fashion. It usually begins with fairly general questions and moves to more specific ones (Bickley, 2017). Questions should initially concentrate on the head, eyes, ears, nose, and throat, and then proceed to focus on the neck, lungs, heart, abdomen, and genitourinary system. The ROS should conclude with asking about the extremities, back, muscles, and joints. Information about the child's developmental status or diet, sleep, and elimination patterns may also be included in the ROS. If questions lead to answers about the history of present illness, or PMH, those answers should be documented in the appropriate section (Bickley, 2017).

📁 *Patient information continued...* The nurse takes Susie Lynn's weight and height. She is 50 pounds and 47 inches tall. She is 3 pounds heavier than her last well child visit a year ago and 2 inches taller. Mary tells the nurse that Susie Lynn has a great appetite and loves to eat most fruit and vegetables but also has a sweet tooth for candy!

QUESTION 8.7 **(Multiple choice)**

The CDC growth reference chart in Figure 8.1 is used to monitor growth of children age 2 to 20 years (CDC, 2017). What percentile does Susie Lynn fall within for both weight and height?

A) 47 inches tall is the 90th percentile for height and 75th percentile for weight at 50 lb.

B) 47 inches tall is the 70th percentile for height and 45th percentile for weight at 50 lb.

C) 47 inches tall is the 50th percentile for height and 35th percentile for weight at 50 lb.

D) 47 inches tall is the 40th percentile for height and 30th percentile for weight at 50 lb.

Answer: A

🦉 **RATIONALE**

Pediatric growth charts are clinical tools that have been used by nurses and other pediatric healthcare providers to monitor the growth of infants, children, and adolescents in the United States since 1977. Growth charts help assess whether a child's growth is adequate. Growth charts are available for weight, height, and BMI. They are not intended to be used as sole diagnostic instruments; instead, they should be used as tools that assist the pediatric healthcare provider to form a complete clinical picture for the child being measured (CDC, 2017). Selecting the correct growth chart for age, sex, and measurement device is essential to the complete assessment of growth (Hockenberry & Wilson, 2017).

Percentiles are the most commonly used clinical indicator to assess the size and growth patterns of individual children in the US. Percentiles rank the position of an individual by indicating what percent of the reference population the individual would equal or exceed. For example, on the height-for-age

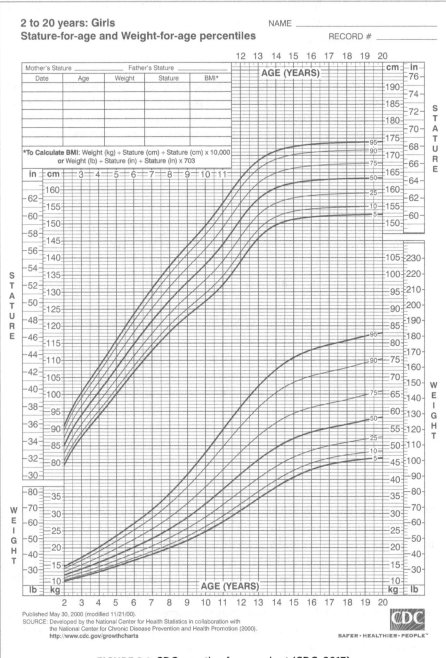

FIGURE 8.1 CDC growth reference chart (CDC, 2017).

growth charts, a 7-year-old boy whose height is at the 25th percentile is as tall as or taller than 25% of the reference population of 7-year-old boys and is shorter than 75% of the 7-year-old boys in the reference population (CDC, 2017). To ensure accuracy when plotting data on the growth chart, the exact chronological age of the child should be used.

QUESTION 8.8 (Multiple choice)

Susie Lynn's grandmother, Mary, asks the nurse what the yearly expected or normal weight gain and increase in height should be for a 6-year-old female.

A) 5 to 6 lb. per year and 4 inches in height for boys and girls

B) 4 to 7 lb. per year and 2 inches in height for boys and girls

C) 1 to 2 lb. per year and 4 to 6 inches in height for boys and girls

D) 4 to 7 lb. per year and 4 inches in height for boys and girl

Answer: B

RATIONALE

Every child's height and weight may vary depending on many different factors, such as genetics; however, an average expected weight gain/year is 4–7 lb. (2–3 kg) for boys and girls, and an average height growth/year is approximately 2 inches (5–6 cm) for boys and girls (Fox, 2020).

QUESTION 8.9 (Multiple response)

Mary explains to the nurse that although Susie Lynn is very active, eats relatively healthily, and presently is at a healthy weight for her age and stature, she worries about her becoming overweight. She states that obesity is a problem in their family, and she fears that Susie Lynn will follow this pattern. Which of the following are guidelines and resources that Mary could implement to prevent Susie Lynn from becoming overweight or obese? *(Select all that apply)*

A) For a 6-year-old child, 90 kcal/kg/day (1,200 to 1,400 cal/day) divided into three meals and two nutritious snacks

B) Limit junk food.

C) Refer to MyPlate for serving sizes, food groups, and recommendations.

D) Encourage families eating together at mealtime.

Answer: A, B, C, D

RATIONALE

In addition to the above guidelines and resources, the AAP (2020) recommends calculating the child's body mass index (BMI)—which is a good indicator of being overweight—beginning at age 2. If your child's BMI is above the 95th percentile for their age, then they have a weight concern that requires further inquiry.

The BMI is calculated from weight and height measurements and is used to judge whether an individual's weight is appropriate for their height. BMI is used to assess underweight, overweight, and risk for overweight in children and teens age 2 to 20 years (CDC, 2017). The BMI is calculated by dividing the child's weight in kilograms by the height in meters squared (kg/m^2; Jarvis, 2016) and is categorized as follows (Hockenberry & Wilson, 2017):

- Normal BMI: Between 18.5 kg/m^2 and 24.9 kg/m^2
- Underweight BMI: Less than 18.5 kg/m^2
- Overweight BMI: Between 25 kg/m^2 and 29.9 kg/m^2
- Obesity (class 1): BMI between 30 kg/m^2 and 34.9 kg/m^2
- Obesity (class 2): BMI between 35 kg/m^2 and 39.9 kg/m^2
- Extreme obesity (class 3): BMI greater than 40 kg/m^2

Those children with BMIs between the 85th and 95th percentiles are considered overweight, and those with a BMI greater than the 95th percentile are considered obese (Hockenberry & Wilson, 2017).

QUESTION 8.10 **(Multiple response)**

When reviewing Susie Lynn's oral hygiene with both her and her grandmother, which of the following educational tips are important to emphasize? *(Select all that apply)*

A) Semiannual dental visits should be adhered to.

B) Regular tooth brushing twice a day

C) Rinsing the mouth twice a day with a strong mouthwash to prevent decay

D) May need fluoride supplements if not in their present water supply

---

Answer: A, B, D

RATIONALE

All the above educational tips are important to emphasize, except rinsing the mouth twice a day with a strong mouthwash to prevent decay. This is not necessary and may be harmful to a child's oral mucosa.

QUESTION 8.11 **(Multiple response)**

In reviewing Susie Lynn's growth and development, which of the following milestones would one expect of a 6-year-old? *(Select all that apply)*

A) Well-established vocabulary

B) Can handwrite simple stories

C) Moves from magical thinking to concrete operations

D) Starts to grasp the concept of time

Answer: A, C, D

RATIONALE

It would be unusual for a child be able to write simple stories until about the age of 10, as most children this age are just beginning to write clearly and formulate simple words independently (Fox, 2020). In addition to the noted developmental milestones of a 6-year-old listed above, the child is also able to begin to understand the feelings of others. They are growing more independent but feel less secure at the same time. They crave affection from parents/caregivers/teachers. Other mastered skills at this age include (Fox, 2020):

- Independent in dressing and hygiene, feeds self, monitoring only as needed
- Can recite address and phone number
- Can draw and copy shapes
- Can draw a man with six parts
- Can print some letters and numbers
- Can articulate needs but may sometimes be incorrect
- Recognizes most letters of the alphabet
- Can define at least seven words
- Can identify some opposites
- Can make decisions using simple logic
- Can balance on each foot for six seconds
- Can heel and toe frontward and backward
- Rides a tricycle without a problem

CHAPTER 8 WORKSHEET

Based on my initial assessment, I thought:

_____

_____

_____

Based on my revised/informed assessment, I now know:

_____

_____

_____

A nursing priority for this patient would be _____

because _____

After completing this chapter, something I have learned is:

_____

_____

_____

After completing this chapter, something I need more clarity on is:

_____

_____

_____

After completing this chapter, something else I want to learn is:

_____

_____

_____

REFERENCES

Ball, J. W., Bindler, R. C., Cowen, K. J., & Shaw, M. R. (2017). *Principles of pediatric nursing: Caring for children* (7th ed.). Pearson Education.

Bickley, L. S. (2017). *Bates' guide to physical examination and history taking.* Wolters Kluwer.

Centers for Disease Control and Prevention. (2017). Clinical growth charts. https://www.cdc.gov/growthcharts/clinical_charts.htm#Set2

Centers for Disease Control and Prevention. (2019). *HPV vaccine schedule and dosing.* https://www.cdc.gov/hpv/hcp/schedules-recommendations.html

Centers for Disease Control and Prevention. (2021). *Influenza (flu) vaccine (inactivated or recombinant): What you need to know.* https://www.cdc.gov/vaccines/hcp/vis/vis-statements/flu.html

Centers for Disease Control and Prevention. (2023). *Recommended child and adolescent immunization schedule for ages 18 years or younger.* https://www.cdc.gov/vaccines/schedules/downloads/child/0-18yrs-child-combined-schedule.pdf

Fox, J. A. (2020). Six year visit: School readiness. In B. Richardson (Ed.), *Pediatric primary care: Practice guidelines for nurses* (4th ed., pp. 139–146). Jones & Bartlett Learning.

Hockenberry, M. J., & Wilson, D. (2017). *Wong's essentials of pediatric nursing.* Saunders.

Jarvis, C. (2016). *Physical examination & health assessment* (7th ed.). Saunders.

The Joint Commission. (2010). *Advancing effective communication, cultural competence, and patient- and family-centered care.* https://www.jointcommission.org/-/media/tjc/documents/resources/patient-safety-topics/health-equity/aroadmapforhospitalsfinalversion727pdf.pdf

Neurological Anomalies

Kristi Maynard, EdD, APRN, FNP-BC, CNE

 CASE STUDY

Patient Presenting With Neurological Changes

- 67-year-old male
- Severe headache, followed by facial droop and loss of speech

T 98.9°F oral	**HR** 112 bpm	**RR** 16	**BP** 187/98	**O2** 98%	**Pain** unable to obtain

Mr. Smith, a 67-year-old male, presents to the emergency department accompanied by his daughter. The patient is obtunded. The patient's daughter reports they were sitting at dinner when her father began complaining of a severe headache. Within a half hour, he began to experience a right facial droop and the inability to speak. Upon discovering him in this state, his daughter immediately called 911, fearing her father was experiencing a stroke.

QUESTION 9.1 (Multiple choice)

An "obtunded" presentation is described as:

A) Restless, agitated with a distracted attention

B) Cannot be aroused; no response to stimuli

C) Decreased alertness with a slowed psychomotor response

D) Prompt response to verbal stimuli; oriented to person, place, and time

Answer: C

RATIONALE

An *obtunded presentation* is a decreased level of alertness with a slowed psychomotor response. Terms such as conscious, confused, delirious, somnolent, obtunded, stuporous, and comatose are used to describe a patient's level of consciousness or state of arousal (Lower, 2002; Tindall, 1990). While familiarity with this terminology is strongly recommended, best practice encourages the ability to describe the observed response to stimuli when documenting. Since terms like *somnolent* and *obtunded* have similar presentations and include a spectrum of responses, the description of the response is a more accurate means to document the level of consciousness. Table 9.1 outlines the terms and descriptions used to identify level of consciousness.

TABLE 9.1 Levels of Consciousness

Level of Consciousness	Description
Conscious	Normal; responds appropriately to questions of orientation
Confused	Impaired thinking and responses; disordered attention along with diminished speed, clarity, and coherence of thought (Adams et al., 1997)
Delirious	Disoriented; restlessness, hallucinations, sometimes delusions; disturbance in attention (reduced ability to direct, focus, sustain, and shift attention) and awareness (American Psychiatric Association, 2013)
Somnolent	Sleepy; excessive drowsiness, difficult to arouse, responds to stimuli in a disorganized manner
Obtunded	Decreased alertness; slowed psychomotor responses
Stuporous	Sleep-like state (not unconscious); little/no spontaneous activity; response with grimace or withdrawal from painful stimuli
Comatose	Cannot be aroused; nonresponsive to verbal or painful stimuli

(Porth, 2007)

You may determine a patient's level of consciousness by how they appear and how they respond to verbal and painful stimuli. Verbal stimulation is achieved when the patient responds to a verbal prompt, even if their response is inappropriate. An example of a verbal prompt may be asking a patient to recite their name or even asking, "Are you OK?" A positive verbal response would include the patient answering a verbal prompt (appropriately or inappropriately), re-directing their gaze toward the person speaking, or opening their eyes. If a patient responds to a verbal stimulus, no painful stimulus is warranted.

Painful stimulation is achieved through methods such as supraorbital pressure, trapezius squeeze, fingernail compression, or sternal rub (Lower, 2002). *Supraorbital pressure* is performed by applying firm pressure with the thumb to the indentation above the eye, toward the nose. This action stimulates the supraorbital nerve (Rank, 2010). The *trapezius squeeze* is, as the name describes, the process of pinching the trapezius muscle between the thumb and forefinger (Lower, 2002). *Fingernail compression* involves the application of pressure directly over the nail bed. Finally, the *sternal rub* involves using the knuckles of the fingers in a grinding pattern on the patient's sternum (Rank, 2010). A positive response would include grimace, eye-opening, verbal response, or movement.

QUESTION 9.2 (Multiple response)

Which of the following subjective information collected during the health history would be considered a risk factor for the development of a cerebrovascular accident (CVA)? *(Select all that apply)*

A) 40 pack-per-year cigarette smoker

B) Uncontrolled hypertension

C) A diet high in protein

D) Father sustained a CVA at age 55

E) Seasonal allergies to pollen

Answer: A, B, D

RATIONALE

It is important to differentiate between subjective and objective information. *Subjective* data are reported by the patient or family. *Objective* information is something that can be observed. It is possible for something to be both subjective and objective. An example would be Mr. Smith's blood pressure. His daughter may report that Mr. Smith has a history of uncontrolled hypertension, which would be a subjective report, but the blood pressure reading of 187/98 is an objective finding as it can be observed and measured. Practice identifying subjective versus objective information in the following exercise.

Place an "X" in the appropriate category for the reported sign/symptom.

	Subjective	Objective
1. Nausea		
2. Shoulder pain		
3. Pulse 84		
4. Cervical spine rotation 70 degrees		

1. Subjective; 2. Subjective; 3. Objective; 4. Objective

The major modifiable risk factors for CVA include:

- Hypertension
- Diabetes mellitus
- Smoking
- Dyslipidemia
- Physical inactivity

A *modifiable risk factor* is a state or condition that can be changed. For example, physical inactivity is a major risk factor for CVA; however, this risk factor can be reduced or eliminated with the implementation of a regular exercise routine such as daily walking. Unmodifiable risk factors are those that cannot be changed. For CVA, these include advanced age (> 80 years), ethnicity and race, male sex, and family history. A combination of two or more risk factors greatly increases the risk of suffering a CVA (National Heart, Lung, and Blood Institute, 2023).

Patient information continued... Mr. Smith's modifiable risk factors include smoking and hypertension:

Smoking: Mr. Smith has a reported history of smoking, with a documented consumption of 40 packs per year.

Pack years are calculated to standardize the manner cigarette smoking is documented. The calculation for pack years is:

Packs of cigarettes smoked per day X number of years the person has smoked.

For example, if a patient smoked one pack of cigarettes a day for 10 years, it would calculate to 10 pack years.

Hypertension: Hypertension is a major modifiable risk factor for CVA development. Mr. Smith had a recorded blood pressure of 187/98 at the time of his event.

Normal blood pressure is a *systolic* (top number) less than 120 and/or a *diastolic* (bottom number) less than 80 (120/80). Numbers greater than 120/80 are "elevated" or "hypertensive" according to the American Heart Association (Whelton et al., 2018). Recognition of normal vital signs is crucial when prioritizing patient care and evaluating risk factors.

Both numbers do not need to be elevated to be classified as hypertensive. If a patient's systolic blood pressure was 146 and diastolic 76, the patient would be diagnosed with systolic hypertension because only the systolic value is elevated. Severe, uncontrolled hypertension increases the risk for a number of conditions including CVA, myocardial infarction, and renal disease.

Considering Table 9.2, how would you classify the Mr. Smith's reported blood pressure?

TABLE 9.2 Stages of Hypertension

Stage	Systolic	Diastolic
Elevated	120–129	< 80
Stage 1	130–139	80–89
Stage 2	140 or higher	90 or higher
Hypertensive crisis	180 or higher	120 or higher

(Whelton et al., 2018)

Answer: Hypertensive crisis

QUESTION 9.3 (Multiple response)

In the absence of verbal responsiveness, which of the following methods could the nurse utilize to assess the patient's pain and level of consciousness? *(Select all that apply)*

A) Revised Nonverbal Pain Scale

B) Apgar Scale

C) Glasgow Coma Scale

D) CAGE Questionnaire

E) Wong-Baker FACES Scale

Answer: A, C, E

RATIONALE

Assessing alertness and pain can be a challenge when caring for a nonverbal patient, but it is critical in providing patient-centered care. The Revised Nonverbal Pain Scale (NVPS), Glasgow Coma Scale (GCS), and Wong-Baker FACES Scale are three validated tools for use with the nonverbal population. The NVPS takes into consideration facial expression, activity or movement, guarding, physiological signs or vital signs, and respiratory status to generate a number representative of the patient's pain score. While this tool was originally developed for use with patients suffering from severe burns, it has been validated for use with any nonverbal population (Kabes et al., 2009).

The Wong-Baker FACES Scale (see Figure 9.1) was developed for use in children to help them express pain. Since its development, it has been integrated into practice as a means to evaluate pain in children and nonverbal patients alike. The scale depicts faces that correlate to the numeric pain scale to assist patients who are unable to meaningfully reply to traditional pain scales.

Patients are asked to point to the face that matches how they are feeling, so even in the absence of verbal expression or comprehension of written words, the patient can select the face that most closely represents what they are feeling (Wong-Baker FACES Foundation, 2016).

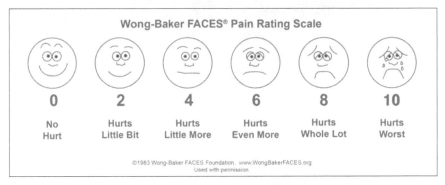

Wong-Baker FACES® Pain Rating Scale

0	2	4	6	8	10
No Hurt	Hurts Little Bit	Hurts Little More	Hurts Even More	Hurts Whole Lot	Hurts Worst

©1983 Wong-Baker FACES Foundation. www.WongBakerFACES.org
Used with permission.

FIGURE 9.1 Wong-Baker FACES Scale.

While the NVPS and Wong-Baker FACES Scale can be used to assess pain, the GCS (see Figure 9.2) is intended to evaluate level of consciousness. The scale measures level of responsiveness in three categories: eye opening, verbal response, and motor response (Teasdale & Jennett, 1974). Each response is scored independently and then cumulatively to determine an overall level of responsiveness. A total score of less than 3 is considered to be completely

Glasgow Coma Scale		
Response	Scale	Score
Eye Opening Response	Eyes open spontaneously	4 Points
	Eyes open to verbal command, speech, or shout	3 Points
	Eyes open to pain (not applied to face)	2 Points
	No eye opening	1 Point
Verbal Response	Oriented	5 Points
	Confused conversation, but able to answer questions	4 Points
	Inappropriate responses, words discernible	3 Points
	Incomprehensible sounds or speech	2 Points
	No verbal response	1 Point
Motor Response	Obeys commands for movement	6 Points
	Purposeful movement to painful stimulus	5 Points
	Withdraws from pain	4 Points
	Abnormal (spastic) flexion, decorticate posture	3 Points
	Extensor (rigid) response, decerebrate posture	2 Points
	No motor response	1 Point
Minor Brain Injury = 13-15 points; Moderate Brain Injury = 9-12 points; Severe Brain Injury = 3-8 points		

FIGURE 9.2 Glasgow Coma Scale scoring.

unresponsive; a total score of 8 or less indicates severe head injury or a coma-tose state. Cumulative scores under 8 are correlated with poor outcomes (Teasdale & Jennett, 1974).

QUESTION 9.4 (Fill in the blank)

List three objective exam findings that would be consistent with a diagnosis of a CVA:

1. _____

2. _____

3. _____

RATIONALE

Objective signs of stroke may include the sudden (generally unilateral) onset of weakness in the extremities, unilateral facial weakness or drooping, aphasia or disrupted speech, vital sign disturbances, vomiting, confusion, and difficulty with balance and ambulation. The Centers for Disease Control & Prevention (CDC) recommends use of the FAST pneumonic for the recognition of common signs of CVA (American Stroke Association, n.d.-b).

F—Face: Ask the person to smile. Does one side of the face droop?

A—Arms: Ask the person to raise both arms. Does one arm drift downward?

S—Speech: Ask the person to repeat a simple phrase. Is the speech slurred or strange?

T—Time: If you see any of these signs, initiate emergency response.

The nursing priority in any emergency scenario is the evaluation and main-tenance of **A**irway, **B**reathing, and **C**irculation, commonly referred to as the **ABCs**. During a CVA, the patient may lose the ability to maintain their air-ways. A decrease in the patient's ability to swallow makes the management of secretions or vomit difficult and may compromise airways. Depending on the severity of the CVA and location of injury within the brain, the patient may have a decrease in their respiratory drive leading to shallow, ineffective, or infrequent breathing patterns (Rochester & Mohsenin, 2002). The nurse must monitor for signs of poor oxygenation such as cyanosis or a blue tint to the lips and mucosa, labored breathing that may include gasping or use of accessory muscles between the ribs leading to retraction, elevated pulse, or a decreased oxygen saturation that may be indicative of impending respiratory failure (CDC, n.d.).

QUESTION 9.5 (Multiple choice)

When assessing for pupillary responsiveness, the nurse observes the following:

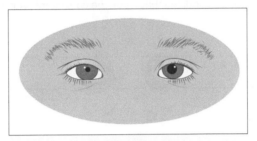

FIGURE 9.3 Pupils.

This would be *best* described as:

A) PERRLA   **B)** Pinpoint   **C)** Anisocoria   **D)** Strabismus

Answer: C

RATIONALE

Anisocoria is described as an uneven dilation of the pupils. This finding may be a normal variant, or it may be indicative of more serious conditions such as CVA (Spencer & Czarnecki, 1983). It may result from increased intracranial pressure.

PERRLA is an acronym to describe the normal function of the pupils in response to light. It stands for: **P**upils, **E**qual, **R**ound, **R**eactive to, **L**ight, and **A**ccommodation. A penlight is used in a dimmed room in an attempt to provoke a response. An expected finding would include the brisk constriction of the pupils in response to light. The response is usually equal in both eyes. An example of pupil sizing can be seen in Figure 9.4.

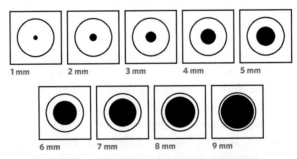

FIGURE 9.4 Measures of pupillary dilation.

The absence of normal dilation may be indicative of a myriad of conditions. When the pupil diameter is less than 2 mm, it is said to be *miotic* (see Figure 9.5). One potential cause of miosis is opioid use. Inversely, *mydriasis* is the abnormal dilation of the pupil and is diagnosed when the diameter of the pupil is greater than 6 mm. Causes of mydriasis may include head injury or use of stimulant drugs such as cocaine. If you recognize an abnormal pupillary reaction, the pupil size and laterality should be documented. An acute change in pupillary response may signify a medical emergency and should be reported promptly to the medical team (Powers et al., 2018).

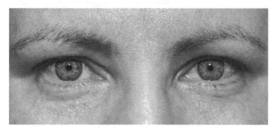

FIGURE 9.5 Miotic pupillary response.

QUESTION 9.6 (Multiple choice)

The nurse recognizes the presence of expressive aphasia during a cerebrovascular accident; this strongly suggests involvement of the _____.

A) Parietal lobe

B) Occipital lobe

C) Temporal lobe

D) Frontal lobe

Answer: D

RATIONALE

Broca's area is a region of the brain located in the frontal lobe that is primarily responsible for speech production. *Broca's aphasia* is a term used interchangeably with *expressive aphasia* to describe the partial or total loss of the ability to produce speech. These patients may be completely unable to formulate words or struggle with word choice. Involvement of Broca's area does not affect the patient's ability to comprehend spoken words; rather, it most frequently disrupts the movements that produce speech.

Wernicke's aphasia, or *receptive aphasia,* is the inability to comprehend speech; it may occur with damage to the parietal and temporal lobe. These patients may have difficulty understanding spoken or written words and may be limited to a basic vocabulary and sentence structure. It is not uncommon for patients with Wernicke's aphasia to use words that are misplaced, repetitive, or inappropriate for what they are attempting to express.

Figure 9.6 illustrates the five major regions of the brain and describes the primary functions of each region.

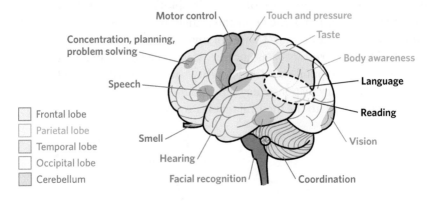

FIGURE 9.6 Brain function by region.

⊕ *Patient information continued...* Upon hospital admission, a CT scan was ordered to determine the cause of Mr. Smith's symptoms. The CT scan confirms the presence of a small hemorrhagic stroke in the frontal lobe. The patient is stabilized and admitted to the neurological intensive care unit for further observation. Two hours after admission to the unit, the nurse caring for Mr. Smith notices his appearance seems rigid, and he begins to experience rhythmic, jerking movements.

QUESTION 9.7 (Multiple choice)

The description of Mr. Smith's seizure activity is best described as:

A) Tonic-clonic seizure

B) Absence seizure

C) Simple focal seizure

D) Atonic seizure

Answer: A

🦉 **RATIONALE**

Tonic-clonic seizures are a type of motor seizure, meaning that they are associated with a physical response paired with an altered mental status. These seizures often appear violent with a sudden onset of rhythmic shaking or convulsing. *Nonmotor seizures* do not include a physical element; instead, the patient's activity may be suspended with the appearance that they are staring off or distracted. This type of seizure is referred to as an *absence seizure* (Epilepsy Foundation, n.d.).

QUESTION 9.8 (Multiple choice)

When prioritizing care of the patient who is actively seizing, the nurse's first action would be:

A) Place a bite block in the patient's mouth

B) Call the physician

C) Ensure patient safety from surrounding objects

D) Assess peripheral blood glucose

Answer: C

RATIONALE

Patient safety is the top nursing priority when a patient is experiencing a seizure. The seizing patient is usually unaware of their surroundings and has no control over the movements of their body. Ensuring the surrounding area is clear of anything that may potentially harm the patient, such as sharp edges, is critical. When possible, the patient's head should be supported with a soft item such as a pillow or blanket (The Nurse Practitioner, 2007). Efforts should be made to prevent the patient from being face down to prevent suffocation. Never place anything in the mouth of the seizing patient because it can be a choking risk. No attempt to restrain the patient or restrict movement should be attempted (The Nurse Practitioner, 2007). While calling for help may be an appropriate action in this scenario, the first priority would be ensuring patient safety.

QUESTION 9.9 (Multiple choice)

The nurse recognizes that a post-CVA seizure is most likely to develop:

A) Within one hour of symptom development

B) Within 24 hours of the cerebrovascular event

C) Within one month

D) Within two weeks

Answer: B

RATIONALE

Approximately 5% of patients who suffer a CVA will develop seizures within the weeks following infarct. The patient is most likely to experience seizure activity within the first 24 hours of the CVA. Seizure activity is more likely in the patient who experienced a hemorrhagic versus ischemic stroke. The presentation of the seizure activity varies greatly among patients and may be an isolated event or lead to a diagnosis of *epilepsy,* a chronic condition involving recurrent seizure activity (American Stroke Association, n.d.-a).

QUESTION 9.10 (Multiple choice)

One week following admission, the nurse reports to Mr. Smith's room to perform her morning assessment. She asks Mr. Smith to smile, lift his eyebrows, and puff out his cheeks. What is the nurse assessing?

A) Cranial nerve VII

B) Verbal comprehension

C) Cranial nerve I

D) Vestibulocochlear function

Answer: A

RATIONALE

Cranial nerves are responsible for the innervation of neurological activity. Nerves can be classified as motor, sensory, or mixed. Each cranial nerve is responsible for a specific function. In the case of Mr. Smith, the inability to perform one of these tasks would be indicative of cranial nerve VII, the facial nerve. See Table 9.3 for a list of cranial nerves.

TABLE 9.3 Cranial Nerves

Number	Name	Function
I	Olfactory	Smell
II	Optic	Sight
III	Oculomotor	Moves eye, pupillary movement
IV	Trochlear	Moves eye
V	Trigeminal	Facial sensation
VI	Abducens	Moves eye
VII	Facial	Facial movement, salivation
VIII	Vestibulocochlear	Hearing, balance
IX	Glossopharyngeal	Taste, swallow
X	Vagus	Heart rate, digestion
XI	Accessory	Moves head
XII	Hypoglossal	Moves tongue

Cranial nerves III, IV, and VI work together to produce the movements of the eye. These movements are known as *extraocular movements* and are tested using the six cardinal fields of gaze. Test the *six cardinal fields of gaze* by having the patient focus on your finger and follow the motion of your finger using only their eyes; no head movement should be involved. The inability to draw or sustain gaze in any direction correlates to dysfunction with either cranial nerve III, IV, or VI. Figure 9.7 illustrates the six fields of gaze and identifies the cranial nerve involved with each movement.

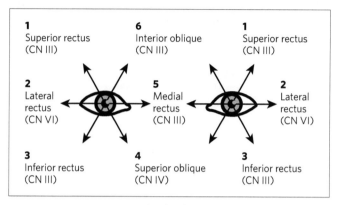

1
Superior rectus
(CN III)

6
Interior oblique
(CN III)

1
Superior rectus
(CN III)

2
Lateral
rectus
(CN VI)

5
Medial
rectus
(CN III)

2
Lateral
rectus
(CN VI)

3
Inferior rectus
(CN III)

4
Superior oblique
(CN IV)

3
Inferior rectus
(CN III)

FIGURE 9.7 Cardinal fields of gaze.

Patient information continued... Mr. Smith has been progressing with his recovery. Today, he will be participating in his first physical therapy session. As they begin, the physical therapist assesses Mr. Smith's strength and sensation. The physical therapist notes the strength in Mr. Smith's right lower leg to be a 2/5 with flexion. He proceeds to assess Mr. Smith's patellar deep tendon reflex on the right side and scores it as a +2. With consideration to Mr. Smith's muscle strength, the therapist decides against performing a Romberg's test.

QUESTION 9.11 (Multiple choice)
When scoring muscle strength, a score of 2/5 indicates:

A) No muscle activation

B) Muscle activation against some resistance

C) Muscle activation with gravity eliminated

D) Trace muscle activation

Answer: C

RATIONALE
The Medical Research Council Manual Muscle Testing Scale is the most commonly used method used to evaluate muscle strength (see Table 9.4). This scale scores muscular response of key muscles on a 0–5 scale. Frequently tested muscles include shoulder abductors, elbow flexors, elbow extensors, wrist extensors, finger flexors, hand intrinsic, hip flexors, knee extensors,

dorsiflexors, great toe extensor, and plantar flexors (Naqvi & Sherman, 2023). Testing different muscles will provide information about the responsiveness of a particular nerve root. For example, when testing elbow strength, you are testing the biceps and triceps muscles, respectively. A poor response from the triceps muscle may indicate disrupted nerve root innervation at the level of C7 in the spinal column.

TABLE 9.4 Muscle Strength Scoring

Medical Research Council Manual Muscle Testing Scale	
Score	Description
0	No muscle activation
1	Trace muscle activation, such as a twitch, without achieving full range of motion
2	Muscle activation with gravity eliminated, achieving full range of motion
3	Muscle activation against gravity, full range of motion
4	Muscle activation against some resistance, full range of motion
5	Muscle activation against examiner's full resistance, full range of motion

(Naqvi & Sherman, 2023)

QUESTION 9.12 (Hotspot)

Place an "X" over the locations of each upper and lower deep tendon reflex.

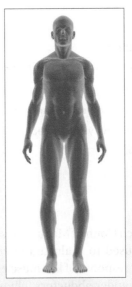

FIGURE 9.8 Anatomic position.

🦉 ANSWER(S)/RATIONALE

Deep tendon reflexes are involuntary muscular movements that are provoked when a specified tendon is struck using a rubber reflex hammer. This involuntary response gives the examiner information about the condition of the muscle's neurological innervation. There are upper and lower sites where deep tendon reflexes can be observed. The five primary reflexes include the biceps, triceps, brachioradialis, patellar, and Achilles (see Figure 9.9).

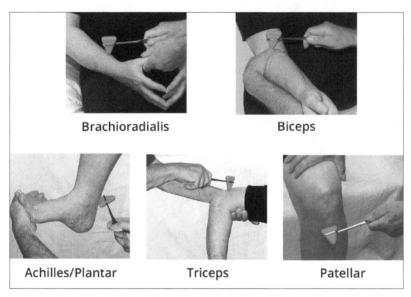

Brachioradialis   Biceps

Achilles/Plantar   Triceps   Patellar

FIGURE 9.9 Reflex sites.

A decreased or absent reflex is classified as *hyporeflexia* and may indicate damage to the nerve root or spinal cord. Inversely, an exaggerated response is termed *hyperreflexia* and might indicate a spinal cord injury. Deep tendon reflexes are scored using a 0–4+ scale (see Table 9.5). Anything from a 1–3+ score may be considered normal with consideration to the patient's previous level of responsiveness; past performance must be compared (if available) when interpreting results. If a patient presents with a patellar reflex of 3+ during their annual exam but had the same response in previous years, it would be considered a normal finding. If the same patient had a 1+ patellar reflex during last year's exam, the examiner might be concerned.

Clonus may be observed with a 4+ response. *Clonus* is the rhythmic, oscillating, stretch reflex that may be observed in motor neuron disease. You are most likely to observe clonus with dorsiflexion of the ankle. It is always an abnormal finding (Zimmerman & Hubbard, 2023).

TABLE 9.5 Deep Tendon Reflex Scoring

Scoring Deep Tendon Reflexes	
Score	Response
0	No response; always abnormal
1+	A slight but definitely present response; may or may not be normal
2+	A brisk response; normal
3+	A very brisk response; may or may not be normal
4+	A tap elicits clonus; always abnormal

(Walker, 1990)

QUESTION 9.13 (Fill in the blank)

During a neurological exam, the nurse asks the patient to stand with both feet together, arms at their sides, and close their eyes. This test is referred to as _____ and tests a patient's _____:

A) Romberg's test; proprioception

B) Phalen's test; level of consciousness

C) Mini-Mental Status Examination; cognition

D) Babinski reflex; pyramidal function

Answer: A

RATIONALE

Romberg's test is performed when the patient stands with both feet together, their arms at their sides, with their eyes closed for 30 seconds. In this position, the nurse is looking for signs of decreased proprioception, which would include swaying or loss of balance. This response would be considered a positive Romberg's test and would indicate vestibular dysfunction (Lanska & Goetz, 2000). When looking to perform Romberg's test, the nurse must evaluate if attempting this exam is safe for the patient. If a patient has difficulty ambulating, has poor muscular strength like Mr. Smith, or is a known fall risk for any reason, they are not an appropriate candidate for this exercise.

The *Mini-Mental Status Examination* (MMSE) is a scripted evaluation commonly used with the elderly to determine the presence of cognitive dysfunction, specifically Alzheimer's disease. The MMSE asks the patient to respond to questions of orientation as well as oral and written activity prompts, including a drawing exercise (see Figure 9.10). The exam is scored out of 30 total points, with 0–17 indicating severe cognitive impairment, 18–23 mild cognitive impairment, and 24–30 no cognitive impairment. Adjustments to scoring may be made for education level and baseline cognitive disturbances (Crum et al., 1993).

Drawing Exercise Mini-Mental Status Exam

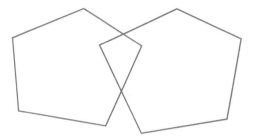

FIGURE 9.10 MMSE drawing exercise.

The *Babinski reflex*, sometimes referred to as the *plantar reflex*, involves the upward stroking motion with a blunt edge on the plantar aspect of the foot (see Figure 9.11). In an adult patient, the outward flaring of the toes indicates a positive Babinski reflex. A positive result may indicate the presence of pyramidal dysfunction or a central nervous system disorder. A positive Babinski reflex is considered normal in children up to 2 years old (Neelon & Harvey, 1999).

Upper motor neuron lesion: Babinski sign

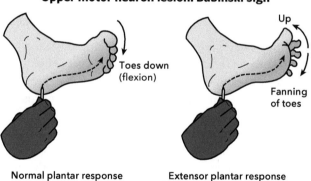

FIGURE 9.11 Babinski reflex.

Patient information continued... Mr. Smith is preparing for hospital discharge following inpatient medical management. As a result of his stroke, he has started an anti-hypertensive regimen including lisinopril and hydrochlorothiazide. Despite intensive physical therapy, Mr. Smith continues to experience weakness in the right upper and lower limbs and expressive aphasia.

QUESTION 9.14 (Fill in the blank)

What subjective information should you, as the discharging nurse, gather from Mr. Smith and his family prior to hospital release?

_____

_____

_____

_____

_____

RATIONALE

The top priority for Mr. Smith's discharge home is safety. Remember, *subjective information* is information that is reported by the patient or their family. Each stroke patient has different discharge needs depending on the severity and location of their CVA. To provide patient-centered care, the nurse needs to gather data on the patient's individual needs, values, health-care beliefs, and health status to develop measurable goals for care. The nurse works as a member of the interdisciplinary team to help identify potential barriers to wellness to meet a patient's short- and long-term health goals.

As the discharging nurse, information concerning the safety and feasibility of the patient returning to his home environment is of vital importance. You might want to know about the layout of the house. Are there stairs? Does he live alone? Will there be someone staying with him during his recovery? Give special consideration to Mr. Smith's aphasia because he may be unable to call for help or explain an emergency. Will he have access to an emergency alert system? With his muscular weakness, will he be able to open pill bottles? Of course, these are only a few examples, but they illustrate the importance of a thorough interview and the breadth of the nurse's role.

CHAPTER 9 WORKSHEET

Based on my initial assessment, I thought:

_____

_____

_____

Based on my revised/informed assessment, I now know:

_____

_____

_____

A nursing priority for this patient would be _____

because _____

After completing this chapter, something I have learned is:

_____

_____

_____

After completing this chapter, something I need more clarity on is:

_____

_____

_____

After completing this chapter, something else I want to learn is:

_____

_____

_____

REFERENCES

Adams, R. D., Victor M., & Ropper, A. H. (1997). Delirium and other acute confusional states. In R. D. Adams, M. Victor, & A. H. Ropper (Eds.)., *Principles of neurology* (6th ed., pp. 431–443). McGraw Hill.

American Psychiatric Association. (2013). *Diagnostic and statistical manual of mental disorders* (5th ed.). Author.

American Stroke Association. (n.d.-a). *Controlling post stroke seizures.* https://www.stroke.org/en/about-stroke/effects-of-stroke/physical-effects-of-stroke/physical-impact/controlling-post-stroke-seizures

American Stroke Association. (n.d.-b). *Learn more stroke warning signs and symptoms.* https://www.strokeassociation.org/en/about-stroke/stroke-symptoms/learn-more-stroke-warning-signs-and-symptoms

Centers for Disease Control and Prevention. (n.d.). *Stroke signs and symptoms.* https://www.cdc.gov/stroke/signs_symptoms.htm

Crum, R. M., Anthony, J. C., Bassett, S. S., & Folstein, M. F. (1993). Population-based norms for the Mini-Mental State Examination by age and educational level. *JAMA, 269*(18), 2386–2391.

Epilepsy Foundation. (n.d.). *Types of seizures.* https://www.epilepsy.com/learn/types-of-seizures

Kabes, A. M., Graves, J. K., & Norris, J. (2009). Further validation of the nonverbal pain scale in intensive care patients. *Critical Care Nurse, 29*(1), 59–66. https://doi.org/10.4037/ccn2009992

Lanska, D. J., & Goetz, C. G. (2000). Romberg's sign: Development, adoption, and adaptation in the 19th century. *Neurology, 55*(8), 1201–1206.

Lower, J. (2002). Facing neuro assessment fearlessly. *Nursing, 32*(2), 58–65. https://doi.org/10.1097/00152193-200202000-00054

Naqvi, U., & Sherman, A. I. (2023). Muscle strength grading. *StatPearls.* https://www.ncbi.nlm.nih.gov/books/NBK436008/

National Heart, Lung, and Blood Institute. (2023). *What is a stroke?* https://www.nhlbi.nih.gov/health-topics/stroke

Neelon, F. A., & Harvey, E. N. (1999). The Babinski sign. *New England Journal of Medicine, 340*(3), 196.

The Nurse Practitioner. (2007). Guide to care for patients: Managing seizures. *The Nurse Practitioner, 32*(5), 19–20.

Porth, C. (2007). *Essentials of pathophysiology: Concepts of altered health states.* Lippincott Williams & Wilkins.

Powers, W. J., Rabinstein, A. A., Ackerson, T., Adeoye, O. M., Bambakidis, N. C., Becker, K., Biller, J., Brown, M., Demaerschalk, B. M., Hoh, B., Jauch, E. C., Kidwell, C. S., Leslie-Mazwi, T. M., Ovbiagele, B., Scott, P. A., Sheth, K. N., Southerland, A. M., Summers, D. V., & Tirschwell, D. L., on behalf of the American Heart Association Stroke Council. (2018). 2018 guidelines for the early management of patients with acute ischemic stroke: A guideline for healthcare professionals from the American Heart Association/American Stroke Association. *Stroke, 49*(3), e46–e99. https://doi.org/10.1161/STR.0000000000000158

Rank, W. (2010). Simplifying neurologic assessment. *Nursing Made Incredibly Easy, 8*(2), 15–19. https://doi.org/10.1097/01.NME.0000368746.06677.7c

Rochester, C. L., & Mohsenin, V. (2002). Respiratory complications of stroke. *Seminars in Respiratory and Critical Care Medicine, 23*(3), 248–260.

Spencer, J. A., & Czarnecki, J. S. (1983). The pupil in stroke. *Canadian Journal of Ophthalmology, 18*(5), 226–227.

Teasdale, G., & Jennett, B. (1974). Assessment of coma and impaired consciousness. A practical scale. *The Lancet, 13*(2), 81–84.

Tindall, S. C. (1990). Level of consciousness. In H. K. Walker, W. D. Hall, & J. W. Hurst (Eds.), *Clinical methods: The history, physical, and laboratory examinations* (pp. 296–299). Butterworth Publishers.

Walker, H. K. (1990). Deep tendon reflexes. In H. K. Walker, W. D. Hall, & J. W. Hurst (Eds.), *Clinical methods: The history, physical, and laboratory examinations* (pp. 365–368). Butterworth Publishers.

Whelton, P., Carey, R., Aronow, W., Casey, D., Collins, K., Dennison Himmelfarb, C., DePalma, S., Gidding, S., Jamerson, K., Jones, D., MacLaughlin, E., Muntner, P., Ovbiagele, B., Smith, S. C., Spencer, C. C., Stafford, R., Taler, S., Thomas, R., Williams, K., Williamson, J., & Wright, J. (2018). 2017 ACC/AHA/AAPA/ABC/ACPM/ AGS/APhA/ASH/ASPC/NMA/PCNA guideline for the prevention, detection, evaluation, and management of high blood pressure in adults: A report of the American College of Cardiology/American Heart Association Task Force on Clinical Practice Guidelines. *Hypertension, 71*(6), 1269–1324. https://www.ahajournals.org/doi/full/10.1161/HYP.0000000000000065

Wong-Baker FACES Foundation. (2016). *Welcome to the Wong-Baker FACES Foundation.* https://wongbakerfaces.org/

Zimmerman, B., & Hubbard, J. B. (2023). Clonus. *StatPearls.* https://www.ncbi.nlm.nih.gov/books/NBK534862/

Cardiovascular and Vascular Anomalies

Kristi Maynard, EdD, APRN, FNP-BC, CNE

CASE STUDY
Patient Presenting With Chest Pain

- 60-year-old male
- Onset of chest pain during activity x one hour
- Arrived by paramedic

T 98.0° F oral	**HR** 90 bpm	**BP** 162/84	**RR** 24	**02** 96%	**Pain** 7/10

Mr. Jones is a 60-year-old male with a history of hyperlipidemia, obesity, and aortic stenosis. He has a 20-pack/year smoking history but quit 10 years ago. He reports the pain started one hour ago and is in the middle of his chest. It started while he was doing work in the yard. The pain moved into his left shoulder, and he states it feels like "pressure." He is sweaty, pale, and appears to be short of breath. His wife called 911, and paramedics arrived shortly after. Mr. Jones is alert and oriented to person, place, and time, but is having difficulty speaking due to severe shortness of breath.

QUESTION 10.1 (Multiple choice)
Considering Mr. Jones's initial presentation, what is his most likely diagnosis?

- **A)** Cerebral vascular accident
- **B)** Myocardial infarction
- **C)** Pulmonary embolism
- **D)** Gastroesophageal reflux disease

Answer: B

RATIONALE
A *myocardial infarction* (MI), or heart attack, is a potentially life-threatening condition affecting over 1.5 million people in the United States every year (Million Hearts, n.d.). As a healthcare professional, it is pivotal that you can recognize the signs and symptoms of MI and intervene appropriately.

Although the other conditions listed may also produce chest pain or vital sign disturbances, Mr. Jones's presentation most closely matches an MI.

Signs and symptoms of MI might include (Heart.org, 2022):

- Chest discomfort usually described as crushing, squeezing, or fullness in the center or left side of the chest
- Pain radiating into one or both arms, the jaw, or the back
- Shortness of breath
- Nausea, vomiting, or diaphoresis (sweating)
- Lightheadedness

These symptoms will vary in presentation and intensity from one patient to the next. Some patients suffering from MI appear to be in acute distress, as is the case with Mr. Jones, while others are unaware they are experiencing an MI at all, which occurs during a silent MI (FamilyDoctor.org, 2023).

Historically, men have received more medical referrals and care for the prevention and treatment of coronary heart disease, the predisposing condition to MI development. In more recent years, there has been a movement to increase education and awareness of women's risk for developing MI. When discussing heart attack risk with female patients, the potential for atypical MI presentation is critical. Women are more likely to experience vague or mild symptoms including:

- Burning sensation in their upper abdomen
- Back pain
- Aching jaw
- Lightheadedness
- Upset stomach
- Sweating

Many times, these symptoms are attributed to other conditions, like indigestion. Heart attacks tend to be more severe in women. In the first year after an MI, women are 50% more likely than men to die from coronary disease or complications (Texas Heart Institute, n.d.).

Patient information continued... Mr. Jones arrives at the emergency department of his local hospital. He already has IV access established from the paramedics. The nurse provides a dose of oral nitroglycerin, starts Mr. Jones on supplemental oxygen via nasal cannula, and administers a dose of IV morphine. The physician has been notified of Mr. Jones's arrival and is on his way from the floor. The nurse proceeds to perform her intake assessment of Mr. Jones.

QUESTION 10.2 (Multiple choice)

When palpating the point of maximal impulse, the nurse appropriately places her fingers on:

A) The left sternal border at the second intercostal space

B) The right sternal border at the fourth intercostal space

C) The midclavicular line at the fifth intercostal space

D) The left sternal border at the third intercostal space

Answer: C

RATIONALE

The *point of maximal impulse* (PMI), or apical pulse, is a palpable landmark that represents the point at which the apex of the heart bounds against the chest wall during contraction. We can predict this landmark will fall at the midclavicular line between the fourth and fifth intercostal space (Gupta & Shea, 2023b). An *intercostal space* is defined as the space between two ribs. Should the PMI be palpated at a different location, it may indicate displacement or enlargement of the heart.

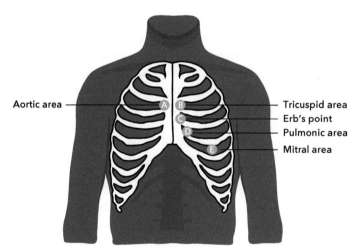

FIGURE 10.1 Cardiac auscultatory locations.

Figure 10.1 represents the anatomical auscultatory locations that are included as part of a comprehensive cardiac exam. When you are auscultating heart sounds, the first thing you are evaluating is the presence of normal heart sounds, the "lub" and the "dub" or S$_1$ and S$_2$. The aortic, tricuspid, pulmonic, and mitral regions each correlate to a heart valve. These specified regions are where sounds from that particular valve are most likely to be accentuated.

Because the aortic and pulmonic valves are located at the base of the heart (remember, when discussing the heart, the base is the top and apex is the bottom), S_2 are heard louder than S_1. The tricuspid and mitral regions are located at the apex of the heart, making S_1 louder than S_2. Erb's point does not correlate with a heart valve but is significant because it is the auscultatory location where S_1 and S_2 will produce equal intensity. Cardiac auscultation should be conducted using both the bell and the diaphragm of the stethoscope to best appreciate both high and low frequency heart sounds. It is imperative to listen for a full minute in each location because not all abnormal heart sounds will be heard in every location (Gupta & Shea, 2023a).

QUESTION 10.3 **(Multiple choice)**

While auscultating in the aortic region, the nurse hears a harsh blowing sound during systole. The nurse attributed this to the patient's history of:

A) Aortic stenosis

B) Hyperlipidemia

C) Mitral regurgitation

D) Myocardial infarction

Answer: A

RATIONALE

The sound described fits the description of the murmur associated with aortic stenosis. A *murmur* is an abnormal heart sound produced by turbulent blood flowing through the valves of the heart. Turbulence may be cause by congenital defect, damage, or hardening of the cardiac valves and can occur in varying degrees (Mayo Clinic, 2022). Some murmurs can be benign while others require medical attention. When describing a murmur, there are seven characteristics to address—each of these descriptors helps to pinpoint the cause, location, and severity of the murmur:

1. Timing
2. Shape
3. Intensity
4. Location
5. Radiation
6. Pitch
7. Quality

Timing

Timing concerns when the murmur occurs in the cardiac cycle. Does it occur during systole or diastole? A murmur is considered *systolic* if the abnormal sound is heard between S_1 and S_2. A murmur is considered *diastolic* if the abnormal sound is heard between S_2 and the subsequent S_1 (Gupta & Shea, 2023b; see Figure 10.2).

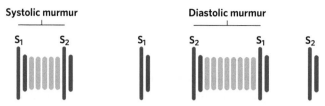

FIGURE 10.2 Describing murmur timing.

Shape

Shape describes the pattern of the sound. Does it remain the same through-out? Does it start strong and then wane? We use musically derived terms such as *crescendo* and *decrescendo* to describe the shape of the murmur.

Intensity

Intensity speaks to the loudness of the murmur (see Table 10.1). With more severe murmurs, a thrill may be present. A *thrill* is a palpable vibration of the chest wall caused by extreme, turbulent blood flow.

TABLE 10.1 Classifying Graded Murmurs

Intensity	Description
Grade I/VI	Barely audible
Grade II/VI	Audible but soft
Grade III/VI	Easily audible
Grade IV/VI	Easily audible with associated thrill
Grade V/VI	Easily audible, with associated thrill, and heard with stethoscope lightly on the chest wall
Grade VI/VI	Easily audible, with associated thrill, and heard with stethoscope off of the chest wall

Location

Location describes the physical location where the murmur was heard. We would use the auscultatory locations previously discussed to describe location.

Radiation

Radiation addresses if the sound is heard in a region other than the primary auscultatory location.

Pitch

Pitch is described as being low, medium, or high.

Quality

Finally, quality has many potential descriptors. Some of the more common include musical, blowing, harsh, or rumbling.

In addition to murmurs, you will auscultate for abnormal heart sounds such as S_3 or S_4, which develop in response to fluid volume overload. In some cases, such as pregnancy, S_3 may be considered a normal variant; however, it can also indicate increased circulatory volume that can be potentially dangerous, as is the case in congestive heart failure.

QUESTION 10.4 (Multiple choice)

When approaching the subjective assessment of chest pain, the nurse utilizes which pneumonic to gather pertinent information?

A) RICE

B) HELP

C) PQRST-U

D) SBAR

Answer: C

RATIONALE

The PQRST-U approach to assessing pain ensures that a comprehensive pain assessment is performed (Crozer Health, n.d.):

P—Provocation/Palliation. What makes the pain better or worse?

Q—Quality. How would you describe the pain?

R—Region or Radiation. Where do you feel the pain? Does it travel anywhere else?

S—Severity Scale. On a scale of 0 to 10, zero being no pain at all and 10 the worst of your life, how would you rate your pain?

T—Timing. When did the pain begin?

U—Understanding. What do *you* think it may be?

QUESTION 10.5 (Multiple response)

Which of the following are evaluated using palpation? *(Select all that apply)*

A) Thrills

B) Lifts

C) Apical pulse

D) Murmur

E) Bruit

Answer: A, B, C

RATIONALE

A *thrill* is a palpable vibration of chest wall that may be caused by turbulent blood flow through the heart. A *lift* may also be known as a *heave* and describes the palpable elevation of the chest wall, usually caused by cardiac enlargement or, in some instances, severe respiratory disease. The *apical pulse*, or PMI, is palpated at the midclavicular line at the fifth intercostal space and represents the region where the apex is closest to the chest wall. A *murmur* and a *bruit* would be assessed using auscultatory techniques (Shea & Gupta, 2023a).

Patient information continued... Based on symptoms, ECG, and lab results, it is determined that Mr. Jones is experiencing an MI, and he is brought to the cardiac catheterization lab. The physician performed an angioplasty and placed a stent to the right coronary artery. The procedure was uncomplicated. Prior to the catheterization he received 325 mg aspirin. During the procedure, he received 1,000 cc normal saline, 6,000 units of heparin, and 90 mg of ticagrelor. He was brought to the cardiac floor following his procedure. He reports pain 2/10 in the left wrist puncture site. A dressing is in place that is clean, dry, and intact. He is placed on telemetry monitor and in sinus rhythm with the following vital signs:

| **T** 98.9°F oral | **HR** 50 bpm | **BP** 122/60 | **RR** 14 | **O2** 99% |

QUESTION 10.6 (Multiple choice)

Mr. Jones's ECG strip is shown in Figure 10.3. Based on this strip, Mr. Jones is determined to have:

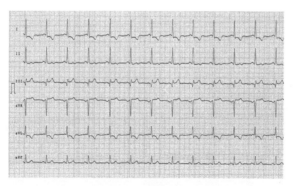

FIGURE 10.3 ECG strip.

A) NSTEMI **C)** Atrial fibrillation

B) STEMI **D)** Bradycardia

Answer: B

RATIONALE

STEMI stands for *ST-elevation myocardial infarction.* If you look at the ECG strip in Figure 10.3, you will notice that the ST segment is elevated from the baseline. MIs classified as STEMIs involve occlusion of large coronary arteries (the blood vessels supplying blood to the heart), and because of this, STEMIs tend to be a more serious MI presentation. *NSTEMIs,* or non-ST-elevation myocardial infarctions, are still serious but generally have better outcomes (Olsen, 2024). In an NSTEMI, the smaller collateral blood supply is occluded, but major vessels are not affected; therefore, there is no ST-elevation apparent on the ECG tracing. *Atrial fibrillation* describes a condition in which the atria of the heart tremor without fully contracting (Mitchell, 2023). *Tachycardia* is the term used to describe an accelerated heart rate above 100 beats per minute. *Bradycardia* is the term to describe a slow heart rate, usually less than 60 beats per minute. Figure 10.4 shows the segments of an ECG.

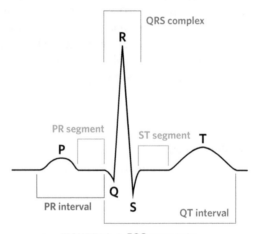

FIGURE 10.4 ECG segments.

QUESTION 10.7 (Multiple choice)

Postoperatively, the nurse evaluates the cardiac catheterization site; it is important to evaluate for bleeding or infection. Based on the nurse's knowledge of pulse points, she proceeds to the _____ to assess the radial pulse.

A) Groin   **B)** Neck   **C)** Foot   **D)** Wrist

Answer: D

RATIONALE

The radial pulse is located on the thumb-side of the wrist. The wrist and groin are common access points for *cardiac catheterization,* a procedure where arterial access is secured and small catheters are inserted into the vasculature to identify and correct blockages. Each pulse point correlates with an underlying artery. We only measure pulse in arteries because they receive high amplitude blood flow every time the heart pumps, causing a measurable pulsation. When evaluating a pulse, we document the pulse rate, regularity, and strength. The *rate* is how many pulsations we feel over the course of a minute. *Regularity* is whether the pulsations you feel occur at a regular or irregular interval. *Pulse strength* describes how strong that pulsation feels against your fingers and is uniformly expressed on a 0–3+ scale shown in Table 10.2.

TABLE 10.2 Pulse Strength

Four-Point Scale	Description
0	Absent
1+	Diminished, weak
2+	Normal
3+	Strong, bounding

As mentioned, there are many pulse points throughout the body. Each location can be seen in Figure 10.5.

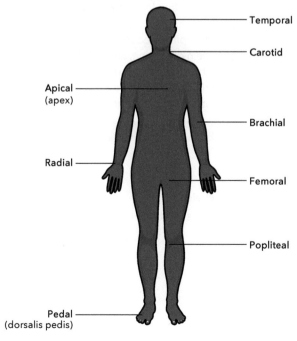

Temporal

Carotid

Apical (apex)

Brachial

Radial

Femoral

Popliteal

Pedal (dorsalis pedis)

FIGURE 10.5 Pulse locations.

QUESTION 10.8 (Multiple choice)

Considering the medications administered during cardiac catheterization, which of the following does the nurse immediately report to the physician?

A) Black, tarry stool

B) Erythema at the IV site

C) Temperature 99.1

D) Headache rated as 3/10

Answer: A

RATIONALE

Black, tarry stool is indicative of gastrointestinal bleeding. During the procedure, Mr. Jones was administered aspirin, heparin, and ticagrelor. Each of these medications is given because of its ability to thin the blood, which decreases clotting risk but increases the risk of minor and major bleeding. Patients who are post-cardiac catheterization or maintained on a blood thinning medication should be monitored for signs of bleeding, including changes to the color of their stool, bleeding mouth or gums, epistaxis (bloody nose), or difficulty controlling bleeding of smalls cuts or wounds (National Institute of Diabetes and Digestive and Kidney Diseases, n.d.).

Patient information continued... The next morning, Mr. Jones reports feeling short of breath while getting out of bed to his chair. His vital signs are shown below. After five minutes sitting in the chair, he reported improvement in symptoms. On exam the nurse notes bilateral 2+ pitting edema in the lower extremities, crackles at lung bases bilaterally, jugular vein distention, and a third heart sound which was not noted by the previous shift. The patient is alert and oriented to person, place, and time with no evidence of dysrhythmia on telemetry monitors. The nurse evaluates the surgical incision, which appears unremarkable.

T 97.8°F oral	**HR** 108 bpm	**BP** 146/92	**RR** 28	**02** 92%	**Pain** 3/10

QUESTION 10.9 (Multiple choice)

Based on Mr. Jones's clinical presentation, the nurse is *most* concerned for:

A) Seizure activity

B) Atrial fibrillation

C) Mitral regurgitation

D) Congestive heart failure

Answer: D

RATIONALE

Congestive heart failure (CHF; see Figure 10.6) occurs when the heart is no longer able to function as an effective pump. CHF may occur for a number of reasons, but damage to the myocardium post-MI is a common cause of heart dysfunction. When the heart is not effectively pumping, fluid backs up into the vasculature, which translates to signs and symptoms of volume overload (Heart.org, 2023).

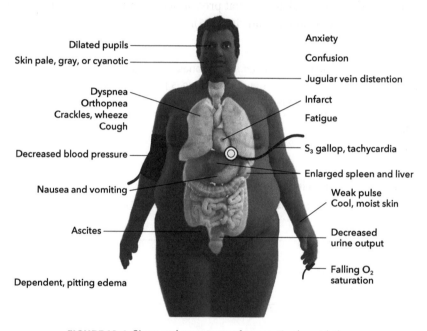

Dilated pupils
Skin pale, gray, or cyanotic
Dyspnea
Orthopnea
Crackles, wheeze
Cough
Decreased blood pressure
Nausea and vomiting
Ascites
Dependent, pitting edema

Anxiety
Confusion
Jugular vein distention
Infarct
Fatigue
S_3 gallop, tachycardia
Enlarged spleen and liver
Weak pulse
Cool, moist skin
Decreased urine output
Falling O_2 saturation

FIGURE 10.6 Signs and symptoms of congestive heart failure.

QUESTION 10.10 (Multiple choice)

While speaking to Mr. Jones, the nurse notices a bulging vessel in his neck. Considering his recent diagnosis of congestive heart failure, the nurse correctly identifies this as:

A) Jugular venous distention

B) Carotid bruit

C) Jugular dissection

D) Lymphadenopathy

Answer: A

RATIONALE

Jugular venous distention (JVD) is a fullness of the jugular vein (located in the neck) that indicates volume overload. When there is venous congestion, pressure in the superior vena cava elevates, causing the bulging appearance of the jugular vein. Although there are methods to formally measure the degree of JVD, you may simply notice the bloated appearance using basic techniques of inspection. Shining a light like a penlight or floor lamp across the neck will help cast shadows that pronounce the appearance of the vessel, making it easier to evaluate (Jarvis, 2016).

Patient information continued... Mr. Jones was stabilized with diuretics, and symptoms of dyspnea and edema resolved. He is preparing to be discharged home with his wife and daily visiting nursing services. He is feeling anxious about leaving the hospital; he feels uncertain about how strong his heart is and fears he may have another heart attack.

QUESTION 10.11 (Fill in the blank)

What are three nursing considerations for Mr. Jones's discharge home?

1. _____

2. _____

3. _____

ANSWERS/RATIONALE

Nursing priorities for Mr. Jones would concern aspects of patient safety, patient education, and the patient's mental health.

QUESTION 10.12 (Multiple choice)

Mr. Jones is struggling with depression and anxiety following his MI. Which of the following statements is *true* regarding mental health assessment?

A) "Mental health is important; however, physical ailments are the priority."

B) "Mental and physical health must be addressed to treat the whole person."

C) "Mental health should only be managed by mental health professionals."

D) "The patient must be stabilized for his heart condition before mental health is assessed."

Answer: B

RATIONALE

Anxiety and depression are common after a patient experiences an unexpected cardiac event, with up to 33% of people reporting mental health symptoms (Pozuelo et al., 2009). As the nurse, it is your responsibility to assess the whole person to deliver patient-centered care focused on the needs of the individual. We also consider the burden of mental stress on the cardiovascular system.

A major recommendation for post-myocardial infarction patients is stress reduction. Undiagnosed or undertreated anxiety and depression contribute to mental stress and may provoke negative physiological responses. Use of an evidence-based depression screening tool to identify patients experiencing depression or at an increased risk is appropriate (Williams, 2011).

Patient information continued... Mr. Jones recovered well following his procedure and was discharged from the hospital. His physician saw him for follow-up and recommended cardiovascular rehabilitation. Mr. Jones began the program, and as his activity increased, he began to report cramping pain in the right calf while walking on the treadmill. The symptoms began after walking for two-and-a-half minutes and were relieved with rest. He also mentions pale discoloration of his right foot that has become more pronounced in recent months. The nurse auscultates the iliac and femoral arteries and notes a bruit in the right femoral location.

QUESTION 10.13 (Multiple choice)

Pain in the legs that begins with physical activity and resolves with rest is known as:

A) Intermittent claudication

C) Charlie horse

B) Venous stasis

D) Vasculitis

Answer: A

RATIONALE

Intermittent claudication is the term used to described pain in the legs that begins with physical activity and resolves with rest. Intermittent claudication is specific to *arterial insufficiency,* a condition where blood supply is restricted as the result of plaque or occlusion. When blood supply to an area, such as the legs, is compromised, the patient will experience pain when there is an increase in oxygen demand. When Mr. Jones begins to walk on the treadmill, the muscles in his legs increase their oxygen demand. The occluded arteries cannot meet this increased demand, and so pain ensues in the oxygen-hungry musculature. When the exercise stops, the pain disappears because the oxygen demand reduces (Teo, 2023).

The symptom of intermittent claudication is unique to arterial disease because arteries carry oxygenated blood. Veins, on the other hand, carry deoxygenated blood back to the heart to re-oxygenate. Veins do not develop plaques in the same manner as arteries, but they can become dysfunctional with conditions such as venous insufficiency. In *venous insufficiency,* the tiny one-way valves that prevent the back flow of blood become damaged, making it difficult for deoxygenated blood to return to the heart. When the venous blood pools, it is known as *venous stasis* and may promote conditions like varicose veins (bulging, painful veins) or venous ulcers (Douketis, 2023).

Both arterial and venous insufficiency are grouped as peripheral vascular diseases. In both cases, ulcer formation and tissue loss are major concerns. If you encounter a vascular ulcer, there are some key differences between venous and arterial ulcerations (see Table 10.3). Discovery of a vascular ulcer requires prompt medical attention and intervention to avoid tissue loss.

TABLE 10.3 Characteristics of Arterial Versus Venous Ulcers

Characteristics	Arterial	Venous
Pain	Sharp, very painful	Cramping, aching (minimal pain)
Pulse	Diminished or absent	Present
Skin	Dry, shiny skin	Reddish-blue in color
Ulcer	Deep	Superficial
Edema	Minimal	Moderate to severe

QUESTION 10.14 (Multiple choice)

The nurse notes auscultation of a bruit in the right femoral region. What is the significance of a bruit?

A) Turbulent or limited blood flow through an artery
B) Normal variant of aging
C) Turbulent or limited blood flow through a vein
D) Increased pulse rate

Answer: A

RATIONALE

A *bruit* is essentially an arterial murmur. The presence of a bruit indicates turbulent blood flowing through an artery. When assessing for bruit, it is best auscultated with the bell of the stethoscope. Bruits can result from arterial narrowing (which is the case in coronary artery disease), or bruits may develop with arterial aneurysm (Lucerna & Espinosa, 2023). An *aneurysm* is a ballooning or out-pouching of an artery. They are most common in the abdominal aorta but can occur anywhere (see Figure 10.7). A ruptured aneurysm is a medical emergency and requires immediate medical attention. Early recognition of an aneurysm may include auscultation of a bruit, the presence of abnormal pulsation in the area of the artery, or reported local pain.

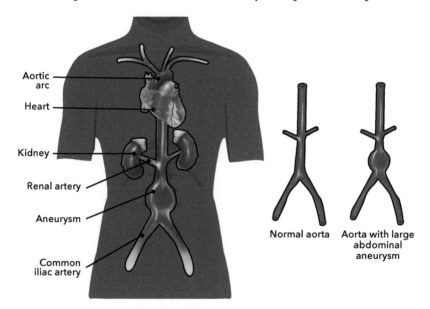

FIGURE 10.7 Abdominal aortic aneurysm.

QUESTION 10.15 (Fill in the blank)

Mr. Jones has now been diagnosed with coronary artery disease, MI, and peripheral vascular disease. What are three risk factors that predisposed him to these conditions?

1. _____

2. _____

3. _____

ANSWER(S)/RATIONALE

Based on Mr. Jones's history, obesity, hyperlipidemia (high blood cholesterol), smoking, and age are all risk factors that may have predisposed him to developing coronary artery disease, MI, and peripheral vascular disease. Major risk factors include hyperlipidemia, high blood pressure, family history of coronary artery disease, diabetes, smoking, men over age 45, postmenopausal women, and obesity (American Heart Association, n.d.).

QUESTION 10.16 (Short answer)

Considering Mr. Jones's risk factors, what patient education will the visiting nurse include to reduce future risk?

_____

_____

_____

_____

CHAPTER 10 WORKSHEET

Based on my initial assessment, I thought:

_____

_____

_____

Based on my revised/informed assessment, I now know:

_____

_____

_____

A nursing priority for this patient would be _____

because _____

After completing this chapter, something I have learned is:

_____

_____

_____

After completing this chapter, something I need more clarity on is:

_____

_____

_____

After completing this chapter, something else I want to learn is:

_____

_____

_____

REFERENCES

American Heart Association. (n.d.). *Coronary artery disease – Coronary heart disease.* https://www.heart.org/en/health-topics/consumer-healthcare/what-is-cardiovascular-disease/coronary-artery-disease

Crozer Health. (n.d.). *PQRST pain assessment method.* https://www.crozerkeystone.org/nurses/pqrst/

Douketis, J. D. (2023, December). Chronic venous insufficiency and post-thrombotic syndrome. *Merck Manual Professional Version.* https://www.merckmanuals.com/professional/cardiovascular-disorders/peripheral-venous-disorders/chronic-venous-insufficiency-and-post-thrombotic-syndrome

FamilyDoctor.org. (2023). *Silent heart attacks.* https://familydoctor.org/condition/silent-heart-attacks/

Gupta, J. I., & Shea, M. J. (2023a, March). Cardiac auscultation. *Merck Manual Professional Version.* https://www.merckmanuals.com/professional/cardiovascular-disorders/approach-to-the-cardiac-patient/cardiac-auscultation

Gupta, J. I., & Shea, M, J. (2023b, March). Cardiovascular examination. *Merck Manual Professional Version.* https://www.merckmanuals.com/professional/cardiovascular-disorders/approach-to-the-cardiac-patient/cardiovascular-examination

Heart.org. (2022). *Heart attack symptoms in women.* https://www.heart.org/en/health-topics/heart-attack/warning-signs-of-a-heart-attack/heart-attack-symptoms-in-women

Heart.org. (2023). *What is heart failure?* https://www.heart.org/en/health-topics/heart-failure/what-is-heart-failure

Jarvis, C. (2016). *Physical examination & health assessment* (7th ed.). Saunders.

Lucerna, A., & Espinosa, J. (2023). Carotid bruit. *StatPearls.* https://www.ncbi.nlm.nih.gov/books/NBK536913/

Mayo Clinic. (2022). *Heart murmurs.* https://www.mayoclinic.org/diseases-conditions/heart-murmurs/symptoms-causes/syc-20373171

Million Hearts. (n.d.). *Costs & consequences.* https://millionhearts.hhs.gov/learn-prevent/cost-consequences.html

Mitchell, L. B. (2023). Atrial fibrillation. *Merck Manual Professional Version.* https://www.merckmanuals.com/professional/cardiovascular-disorders/arrhythmias-and-conduction-disorders/atrial-fibrillation

National Institute of Diabetes and Digestive and Kidney Diseases. (n.d.). *Symptoms & causes of GI bleeding.* https://www.niddk.nih.gov/health-information/digestive-diseases/gastrointestinal-bleeding/symptoms-causes

Olsen, N. (2024). *NSTEMI: What you need to know.* https://www.healthline.com/health/nstemi

Pozuelo, L., Tesar, G., Zhang, J., Penn, M., Franco, K., & Jiang, W. (2009). Depression and heart disease: what do we know, and where are we headed?. *Cleveland Clinic Journal of Medicine, 76*(1), 59–70. https://doi.org/10.3949/ccjm.75a.08011

Teo, K. K. (2023). Peripheral arterial disease. *Merck Manual Professional Version.* https://www.merckmanuals.com/professional/cardiovascular-disorders/peripheral-arterial-disorders/peripheral-arterial-disease?query=intermittent%20claudication

Texas Heart Institute. (n.d.). *Women and heart disease.* https://www.texasheart.org/heart-health/heart-information-center/topics/women-and-heart-disease/

Williams, R. B. (2011). Depression after heart attack: Why should I be concerned about depression after a heart attack?. *Circulation, 123*(25), e639-e640.

CHAPTER 11

Respiratory Anomalies

Andrea Adimando, DNP, MSN, MS, APRN, PMHNP-BC, BCIM

 CASE STUDY

Patient Presenting to Clinic With Shortness of Breath

- 62-year-old female
- History of shortness of breath x 18 months
- History of cough x nine weeks
- Vital signs not yet obtained

Mrs. Brown, a 62-year-old African American woman, comes to your clinic seeking medical attention for increasing shortness of breath on exertion for the past 18 months, and especially today, as well as a cough that has been present for approximately nine weeks. She used to walk 18 holes of golf with her husband every Saturday, but over the last six months has had to use a golf cart due to fatigue and shortness of breath. She initially attributed this change to aging but is worried something more may be going on.

Based on the electronic health record, during the past year, she had three trips to the emergency department and was diagnosed with acute bronchitis. Her primary care provider felt she had developed a case of mild asthma and provided an inhaler for her to use as needed. She has not used the inhaler much because she feels it makes her anxious and does not provide much relief from her symptoms. She smoked 1.5 packs per day for about 17 years but stopped 18 years ago. Her husband smokes cigars in the home two to three times per week. No other significant medical history is reported or noted in her chart.

Family history is significant: Her biological father died of emphysema at age 78 after smoking for 52 years, and her mother is currently living, age 82, with end-stage renal failure and a 40-year history of hypertension. Her maternal grandmother and grandfather both smoked and both died of myocardial infarction. Her paternal grandparent history is unknown.

QUESTION 11.1 (Multiple choice)

Based on this client's history, how many "pack years" of smoking would you record in the medical record?

A) 17 **B)** 18 **C)** 25.5 **D)** 35

Answer: C

RATIONALE

Pack years are calculated by multiplying the number of packs per day that the individual smoked by the number of years the individual smoked. In this case, 1.5 packs per day × 17 years = 25.5 pack years. Pack years is a common term used in medical and nursing charting and helps to quantify the length and amount of damage that the lungs may have endured during the period of smoking.

QUESTION 11.2 (Fill in the blank)

How would you describe the position of the patient seen in Figure 11.1?

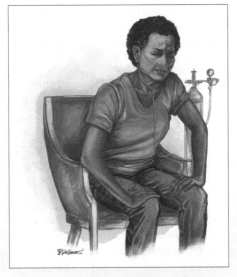

FIGURE 11.1 Patient in respiratory distress.

Answer: Tripod position or tripoding

RATIONALE

Patients with breathing difficulties in advanced lung disease will often assume a tripod position—leaning forward with hands on knees—to force the diaphragm down and reduce the work of breathing (Jarvis, 2020).

Patient information continued... On exam, Mrs. Brown reports feeling short of breath while sitting on the exam table, and she has a capillary refill of four seconds. Some of her fingertips and toenail beds have a slight blue hue, and her face appears pale. She is sitting, leaning forward with her hands on her knees, which she reports is the most comfortable position for her to be in at this time. She denies pain, though her chest feels "uncomfortably tight" most days. She is intermittently coughing throughout the interview, and the cough is sometimes productive, producing thick white sputum at times. Auscultation shows wheezes bilaterally, especially in the right middle lobe and left lower lobe.

T 98.9°F oral	**HR** 98 bpm	**BP** 127/88	**RR** 22	**O2** 92%	**Pain** 0/10

QUESTION 11.3 (Short answer)

List at least three important signs and/or symptoms, current or previous, or important pieces of her history related to Mrs. Brown's respiratory system that would be important pieces of data for the nurse to consider and record to support her assessment and eventual diagnoses by the provider:

_____

_____

_____

_____

_____

QUESTION 11.4 (Categorizing signs and symptoms)

Considering your signs and symptoms listed above, circle the ones that are objective pieces of data, and underline the pieces that are subjective pieces of data.

Answer(s): *Subjective data* come from the client's point of view ("symptoms"), including her perceptions and concerns. *Objective data* are observable and measurable data ("signs") obtained through observation, physical examination, and laboratory and diagnostic testing. Some symptoms can be either subjective or objective, depending on whether they are reported by the patient or witnessed/verifiable by provider.

Subjective data include:

- Shortness of breath on exertion for past 18 months
- Fatigue during usual activities, requiring assistance
- Chest tightness
- Asthma inhaler unhelpful and barely used
- Cough present for approximately nine weeks
- 25.5 pack year history
- Two to three times weekly exposure to unfiltered cigar smoke

Objective data include:

- Vital signs, especially her respiratory rate (RR), which is notably high
- Diagnosed with acute bronchitis 3x in past 12 months (verified by EHR, so objective in this case because it can be confirmed)
- Cyanosis of nailbeds
- Productive cough (objective here because witnessed by the RN during assessment)
- Tripod position
- Pallor in face
- Wheezes heard bilaterally on auscultation

QUESTION 11.5 (Hotspot)

In Figure 11.2, place an X on the spot where the nurse would auscultate the right middle lobe (the answer is in Figure 11.3):

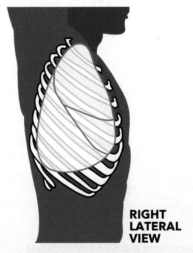

RIGHT
LATERAL
VIEW

FIGURE 11.2 Place an X where you think the right middle lobe would best be auscultated.

Answer:

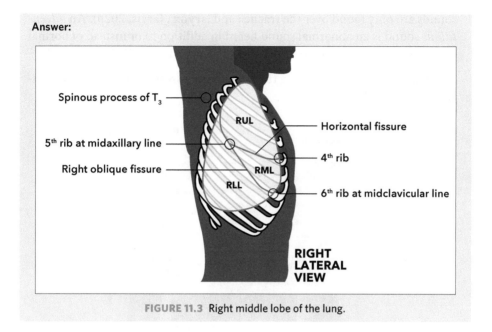

Spinous process of T₃

5ᵗʰ rib at midaxillary line

Right oblique fissure

RUL

Horizontal fissure

4ᵗʰ rib

RML

RLL

6ᵗʰ rib at midclavicular line

RIGHT LATERAL VIEW

FIGURE 11.3 Right middle lobe of the lung.

RATIONALE

The right middle lobe can best be auscultated close to the nipple. Though exact positioning can vary by size and condition of the individual, the right middle lobe generally spans from the fourth intercostal space to the sixth rib, in between the anterior axillary line and the mid-clavicular line (Jarvis, 2020).

QUESTION 11.6 (Multiple choice)

What type of breath sounds should the nurse expect to hear in this region in a healthy individual?

A) Vesicular

B) Bronchovesicular

C) Bronchial

D) Adventitious

Answer: A

RATIONALE

Vesicular breath sounds, which are low-pitched, soft breath sounds, are found over peripheral lung fields. *Bronchovesicular* breath sounds are found posteriorly in the region between the scapulae and anteriorly bordering the sternum between the first and third intercostal space. *Bronchial* breath sounds are only found over the trachea and larynx (Jarvis, 2020). An *adventitious* sound is an abnormal sound heard in addition to or instead of normal lung sounds (such as wheezes or crackles; Zimmerman & Williams, 2023).

All breath sounds heard during the lateral lung assessment would be vesicular (see Figure 11.4).

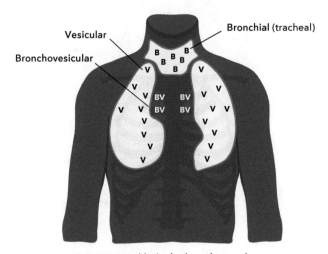

FIGURE 11.4 Vesicular breath sounds.

QUESTION 11.7 (Multiple choice)

Though the nurse will not be diagnosing this patient today, they will be collecting subjective and objective assessment data about this patient, which will help the diagnostic healthcare provider determine the specific diagnosis. The nurse anticipates that, based on the cluster of symptoms, the patient may meet criteria for:

A) Severe asthma

B) Respiratory syncytial virus

C) Chronic obstructive pulmonary disease (COPD)

D) Raynaud's syndrome

Answer: C

RATIONALE

COPD is an inflammatory lung disease that causes some form of obstruction to proper air exchange in the lungs. The most common manifestations of COPD are emphysema and chronic bronchitis. With emphysema, as with chronic bronchitis, the bronchioles are inflamed, and in emphysema the alveoli are damaged from chronic hyperinflation, which impedes airflow to and from the alveoli of the lungs (Jarvis, 2020). This patient is likely suffering from chronic bronchitis, given her:

- Smoking history
- Frequent, productive cough
- History of frequent bronchitis diagnoses
- Signs of obstructed airflow, which include:
  - Cyanosis
  - Pallor
  - Fatigue
  - Shortness of breath, with and without exertion
  - Tripod positioning

The patient's chronic cough is related to excess mucus production, which is a result of the inflammation and narrowing of the bronchial tubes (see Figure 11.5). The cough is an attempt by the body to clear the airways for improved air exchange (Mayo Clinic, 2020).

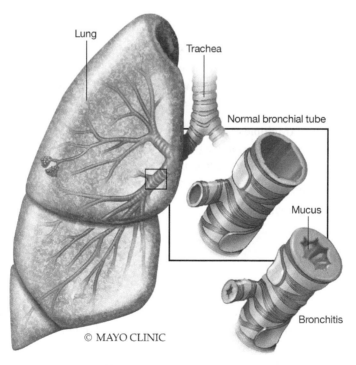

© MAYO CLINIC

FIGURE 11.5 Normal bronchial tubes vs. bronchial tubes in bronchitis.
Used with permission of Mayo Foundation for Medical Education and Research. All rights reserved.

QUESTION 11.8 (Short answer)

Based on what you now know about COPD and about this client, what are her known risk factors for this disease?

_____

_____

_____

_____

_____

 ANSWER(S)/RATIONALE

- 25.5 pack year smoking history
- Two to three times weekly exposure to cigar smoke
- Immediate family history of COPD
- Exposure to secondhand smoke as a child
- Age > 40, as this condition develops gradually over time (Mayo Clinic, 2020; National Heart, Lung, and Blood Institute, 2023)

QUESTION 11.9 (Multiple response)

What type of breath sounds might the nurse be likely to hear in this patient, given what you know so far? *(Select all that apply)*

A) Diminished breath sounds   **D)** Crackles

B) Increased breath sounds   **E)** Friction rub

C) Wheezes   **F)** Rhonchi

Answer(s): A, C, F

RATIONALE

Chronic bronchitis is a condition that is characterized by inflammation in the bronchial tubes, which impairs airflow in and out of the lungs. This can lead to wheezes, which are produced by narrowing of these airways. This can also produce *rhonchi,* which are low-pitched wheezing sounds that typically happen on inspiration, as a result of narrowing of the bronchial tubes either from mucus production or inflammation. Breath sounds may be diminished (or decreased) due to impediments in airflow as previously described. (See Table 11.1 for an overview of adventitious breath sounds.)

TABLE 11.1 Adventitious Breath Sounds

Sound	Description/Cause
Crackles (rales)	Sound description: fine, brief, and discontinuous
	Caused by air passing through fluid or mucus in the small airways and alveoli
	Heard in bases of the lungs
Gurgles	Sound description: low-pitched rattle
(rhonchi)	Caused by air moving the secretions in larger airways
	Heard diffusely over the lungs, but may be louder over the trachea and bronchi
Friction rub	Sound description: a harsh grating or creaking sound
	Caused by inflammation of the pleural tissue
	Heard over the affected area
Wheeze (on exhalation)	Sound description: high-pitched squeaking, musical quality
	Caused by air passing through constricted bronchus
	Heard throughout lung fields

QUESTION 11.10 (Short answer)

What is meant by the term *barrel chest*, and how would the nurse determine whether this patient presented with this characteristic? Write your answer in the space below:

_____

_____

_____

_____

ANSWER/RATIONALE

When assessing a patient, a nurse should always pay attention to the anterior-posterior (A-P) diameter as compared to the transverse diameter of the thoracic cage. In a healthy individual, the ratio of A-P to transverse diameters should be at or very close to 1:2. In a person with COPD, the lungs are chronically hyperinflated, causing the A-P diameter to increase and bringing the ratio closer to 1:1 (see Figures 11.6 and 11.7).

The costal angle—another important characteristic for the nurse to assess during a respiratory assessment—will also be greater than the 90 degrees that is considered normal. This is especially true in emphysema, where the lungs are unable to expel air adequately, leading to chronic hyperinflation. It can also happen in severe, restrictive conditions such as chronic asthma, where the narrowing of the airways contributes to hyperinflation of the lungs (Jarvis, 2020). This ratio is an important factor in not only formulating a diagnosis of COPD but also in determining the chronicity of the condition. The longer the person has been symptomatic, the more pronounced this ratio difference will be.

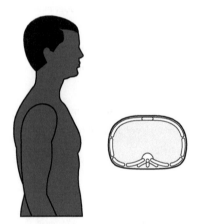 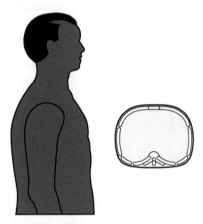

FIGURE 11.6 **Typical chest:** A-P diameter is less than transverse diameter, approximately at a 1:2 ratio.

FIGURE 11.7 **Barrel chest:** Ribs become more horizontal, and A-P transverse diameter is closer or equal to 1:1.

📁 *Patient information continued...* After a thorough review of all the subjective and objective assessment data collected by the RN, as well as a comprehensive history and physical exam, the primary care provider diagnoses the patient with chronic bronchitis, a form of COPD. The primary care provider requests that the nurse provide counseling for the patient on the ramifications of this diagnosis in terms of preventing worsening, comfort measures/alleviating symptoms, and empowering the patient to identify when it is appropriate to seek more emergent care.

QUESTION 11.11 (Short answer)

What are some ways the patient can increase comfort, decrease work of breathing, and alleviate her symptoms of COPD?

_____

_____

_____

_____

 ANSWER(S)/RATIONALE

Positioning:

- Utilize tripod position whenever indicated. This will force the diaphragm to move downward, allowing the lungs to expand more easily and relaxing the musculature around them.
- If patient becomes fatigued during activities, suggest supporting arms by resting elbows on a surface to minimize muscle/energy expenditure in this area of the body (Bauldoff, 2012).

Rest/relaxation:

- To conserve energy and reduce fatigue, patients should be encouraged to pace themselves, taking frequent rest breaks and perhaps breaking down larger activities into smaller steps. Assistive devices such as walkers may be necessary, or in the case of our patient, encouraging her to continue to use the golf cart during her leisure golfing activities (vs. attempting to walk the course).

Breathing techniques to improve airflow:

- Pursed lip breathing can reduce respiratory rate and improve exhalation efficiency.
- Slow, controlled exhalations can help to expel any trapped air that may be stuck in the inflamed bronchioles and prevent further trapping.

Avoid triggers:

- These include environmental triggers such as cigarette/cigar smoke (particularly for our patient), allergens, harsh chemicals, and poor-quality air (such as in large cities or some foreign countries).
- This also includes physiological triggers such as stress or strenuous exercise.

QUESTION 11.12 (Short answer)

When providing care for this patient, what warning signs that may indicate a need to seek care should the nurse teach the patient? Write your answer in the space below:

_____

_____

_____

_____

ANSWER/RATIONALE

The following are some possible answers to the question above, as they all likely indicate that the patient should seek medical care:

- New-onset *cyanosis* (bluish tint) of the core or body extremities
- A sudden increase in shortness of breath
- Dizziness
- Noticeable increase in mucus production or change in color of mucus
- Increased or sudden swelling of the extremities
- Fever
- Shallow or rapid breathing

QUESTION 11.13 (Multiple choice)

When discussing long-term considerations for care for the patient with COPD, which of the following statements by the patient indicates a need for further education?

A) "I will make every effort to quit smoking to preserve my lung function."

B) "I expect a full recovery in six months to one year."

C) "Adhering to my prescribed medications will reduce my symptoms and exacerbations."

D) "I should report any increase in symptoms immediately to my healthcare provider."

Answer: B

RATIONALE

COPD is a chronic and irreversible condition; however, it is preventable through health and lifestyle modifications. It is important to educate your patients on their risk factors for COPD prior to the development of the disease and to assist in any way possible with their modifications of these risk factors. These include, but are not limited to, avoiding environmental toxicants such as chemicals and chemical dust, quitting smoking, and avoiding secondhand smoke and other forms of air pollution (Centers for Disease Control and Prevention, 2023).

Patients can live with COPD for many years with proper management. It is the RN's role to carefully monitor the patient for signs of COPD worsening and to provide education regarding prevention and maintenance of COPD at every visit or hospitalization.

Patient information continued... Mrs. Brown returns to the clinic two months later with complaints of a cough productive for thick, brown sputum, a low fever of 101.2, shortness of breath, and malaise. After auscultating the lungs, percussing the lung fields, and performing tactile fremitus, the primary care provider suspects pneumonia. Vital signs include the following:

T 101.2°F oral	**HR** 100 bpm	**BP** 146/88	**O2** 94%

QUESTION 11.14 (Multiple choice)

Percussion of lung fields affected by pneumonia will likely produce a _____ sound.

A) Resonant

B) Hyper-resonant

C) Tympanic

D) Dull

Answer: D

RATIONALE

Percussion is an assessment technique that allows the examiner to determine tissue or structural density. To perform percussion, place the middle finger firmly over the chest wall and tap over the distal interphalangeal joint with the middle finger of the opposite hand. This action will produce a sound. We expect percussion of healthy lung tissue to have a resonant quality because healthy lungs are filled with air. In the case of pneumonia, a section of the lung has become infiltrated (filled) with fluid, thereby increasing the density of the structure. This change in density will alter the quality of lung field percussion and produce a dull sound (Jarvis, 2020).

QUESTION 11.15 (Multiple choice)

Which of the following correctly describes the procedure for evaluating tactile fremitus?

A) Place the ulnar aspect of the hands on the wall of the chest and have the patient say "99."

B) Place the stethoscope on the lateral chest wall and have the patient say "blue moon."

C) Instruct the patient to take a deep breath and force a cough while auscultating the lung fields.

D) Using the thumbs, pinch the skin of the back at the level of T10 and instruct the patient to take a deep breath.

Answer: A

RATIONALE

Tactile fremitus is an assessment technique that compares vibrations through the lung fields. For the tactile variant, the examiner places the ulnar aspects of the hand on the posterior and/or anterior lung fields while asking the patient to say "99." The vocal expression causes vibrations through the air-filled lung. If vibrations are felt equally on either side, it is considered a normal finding. If there is a unilateral increase or decrease in the perceived frequency of vibration, the examiner may suspect consolidation or infiltrate in the affected lung field (Jarvis, 2020).

Use of the stethoscope to evaluate the transmission of voice is known as *vocal fremitus*. Placing the fingers at the level of T10 and instructing the patient to take a deep breath is evaluating for equal lung expansion. If each hand rises equally, the lungs are filling to a similar capacity. If this exam were noted to be unequal, the examiner may be concerned for conditions of restrictive lung disease or lung collapse (Jarvis, 2020).

QUESTION 11.16 (Multiple choice)

After a physical exam, the primary care provider has a high suspicion for pneumonia. What follow-up exam does the nurse anticipate to confirm the diagnosis?

A) Chest MRI

B) Incentive spirometry

C) Thoracentesis

D) Chest X-ray

Answer: D

RATIONALE

A standard chest X-ray is usually sufficient to confirm the presence of a pulmonary infiltrate. On occasion, small or early infiltrations may not be seen on an X-ray, and a CT scan is indicated (Wootton & Feldman, 2014).

Patient information continued... A chest X-ray confirms Mrs. Brown has bilateral lower lobe pneumonia. The primary care provider recommends she be admitted for treatment secondary to her low oxygen saturation and history of COPD. She is hospitalized for six days while completing IV antibiotics and nebulized breathing treatments. On the seventh day, it is determined she is well enough to return home on supplemental oxygen.

QUESTION 11.17 (Short answer)

Considering Mrs. Brown's recent illness and comorbidities, what teaching should the nurse include during discharge to improve patient safety and wellness?

_____

_____

_____

_____

ANSWER/RATIONALE

There are many possible answers here, but some things you might want to focus on for this particular patient include:

- Safe use of oxygen at home, including keeping oxygen away from stoves (gas, wood, or fireplaces) or any other potential igniters

- Teaching the patient how to self-monitor oxygenation with signs such as delayed capillary refill, oxygen saturation (if a home monitoring device is available), or cyanosis

- Teaching the patient comfort measures to improve oxygenation, such as elevating the head of the bed and/or sleeping on more than one pillow

- Teaching the patient what signs would warrant a call to the doctor vs. a trip to the emergency department vs. no action, based on the discharge instructions of the physician or licensed independent practitioner (LIP)

QUESTION 11.18 (Fill in the blank)

Based on the patient's clinical presentation, what are three nursing priorities for this patient's care?

1. _____

2. _____

3. _____

 ANSWER(S)/RATIONALE

There are several possible answers here, such as:

- Maintaining a patent airway
- Monitoring for and maintenance of regular rate of breathing, decreased work of breathing, and oxygen saturation level, as per LIP orders
- Education for preventing return to hospital and for improved management of underlying conditions
- Ensuring the patient has adequate follow-up with appropriate providers and a social support system to help manage chronic and acute illnesses

CHAPTER 11 WORKSHEET

Based on my initial assessment, I thought:

_____

_____

_____

Based on my revised/informed assessment, I now know:

_____

_____

_____

A nursing priority for this patient would be _____

because _____

After completing this chapter, something I have learned is:

_____

_____

_____

After completing this chapter, something I need more clarity on is:

_____

_____

_____

After completing this chapter, something else I want to learn is:

_____

_____

_____

REFERENCES

Bauldoff, G. S. (2012, Aug. 11). When breathing is a burden: How to help patients with COPD. *American Nurse Today.* https://www.americannursetoday.com/when-breathing-is-a-burden-how-to-help-patients-with-copd-2/

Centers for Disease Control and Prevention. (2023). *Chronic obstructive pulmonary disease (COPD).* cdc.gov/copd/index.html

Jarvis, C. (2020). *Physical examination and health assessment* (8th ed.). Saunders.

Mayo Clinic. (2020). *COPD.* https://www.mayoclinic.org/diseasesconditions/copd/symptoms-causes/syc-20353679

National Heart, Lung, and Blood Institute. (2023). *What is COPD?* https://www.nhlbi.nih.gov/health-topics/copd

Wootton, D., & Feldman, C. (2014). The diagnosis of pneumonia requires a chest radiograph (x-ray)—yes, no or sometimes? *Pneumonia, 5,* 1–7. https://doi.org/10.15172/pneu.2014.5/464

Zimmerman, B., & Williams, D. (2023). Lung sounds. *StatPearls.* https://www.ncbi.nlm.nih.gov/books/NBK537253/

CHAPTER 12

Gastroenterological Anomalies

Tammy Lo, MSN, APRN, ACNP-BC

CASE STUDY

Patient Presenting to the ED With GI Distress

- 52-year-old female
- Reports abdominal discomfort for "quite some time"

T 98.6°F oral	HR 72 bpm	BP 94/46	RR 16	O2 99%	Pain 7/10

Mrs. Johnson is a 52-year-old female who presented to the emergency department accompanied by her daughter with complaints of yellowing of skin, dark urine, and abdominal bloating and fullness. She reports experiencing intermittent abdominal discomfort for quite some time but has not followed up with her primary care provider. She admits to significant alcohol use.

QUESTION 12.1 (Multiple choice)

The mnemonic "PQRST" for assessing pain stands for:

A) Potability, Quantification, Region, Severance, and Temperance

B) Pacification, Quarantine, Resistance, Somnolence, and Time

C) Provocation, Quality, Radiation, Severity, and Time

D) Palliation, Quiescence, Roaming, Sequencing, and Transplantation

Answer: C

RATIONALE

Pain is subjective and can vary with different disease states. Therefore, an accurate description of pain is critical to gather more information about the problem, and it can be vital in determining the appropriate treatment and response. When assessing for pain, "PQRST" is a commonly used mnemonic, standing for (Jarvis, 2012):

Provocation or Palliation

Questions that may be helpful include: What makes the pain worse? Does movement, palpation, laughing, running, or coughing provoke the pain? What makes the pain better? Were any medications used to help alleviate the pain?

Quality

Questions assessing what the pain feels like can be helpful in determining the cause of the pain. Is the pain sharp and stabbing or dull and vague? Is there a tingling or burning sensation or a crushing, vice-like quality?

Region or Radiation

These questions assess the area of the body in which the pain is located and whether the pain is localized or travels (or radiates) to other areas of the body. Example questions include: Where is the pain located? Does the pain travel anywhere?

Severity

These questions assess how mild or severe the pain is. The Numeric Rating Scale is a commonly used tool, requiring the patient to rate the pain on a defined scale (see Figure 12.1). The scale ranges from 0 to 10, with 0 representing no pain and 10 representing the worst pain imaginable. Another validated scale that many patients favor is the Mankoski Pain Scale, as shown in Table 12.1 (Douglas et al., 2014).

Time

These questions assess for duration and chronicity. Example questions include: When did the pain begin? Is the pain constant or intermittent? How long does the pain last?

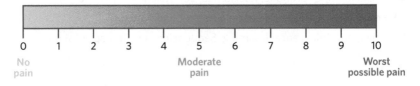

FIGURE 12.1 The Numeric Rating Scale (McCaffery & Beebe, 1989).

TABLE 12.1 The Mankoski Pain Scale

Numerical Pain Rating	Pain Description	Action Required
0	Pain-free	No medication needed.
1	Very minor annoyance—occasional minor twinges	No medication needed.
2	Minor annoyance—occasional strong twinges	No medication needed.
3	Annoying enough to be distracting	Mild painkillers are effective (aspirin, ibuprofen).
4	Can be ignored if you are really involved in your work, but still distracting	Mild painkillers relieve pain for 3-4 hours.
5	Can't be ignored for more than 30 minutes	Mild painkillers reduce pain for 3-4 hours.
6	Can't be ignored for any length of time, but you can still go to work and participate in social activities	Stronger painkillers (codeine, hydrocodone) reduce pain for 3-4 hours.
7	Makes it difficult to concentrate and interferes with sleep, but you can still function with effort	Stronger painkillers are only partially effective. Strongest painkillers relieve pain (oxycodone, morphine).
8	Physical activity severely limited; you can read and converse with effort; nausea and dizziness set in as factors of pain	Stronger painkillers are minimally effective. Strongest painkillers reduce pain for 3-4 hours.
9	Unable to speak; crying out or moaning uncontrollably—near delirium	Strongest painkillers are only partially effective.
10	Unconscious; pain makes you pass out	Strongest painkillers are only partially effective.

(Mankoski, 2000)

QUESTION 12.2 (Fill in the blank)
List the nine regions of the abdomen:

1. _____

2. _____

3. _____

4. _____

5. _____

6. _____

7. _____

8. _____

9. _____

ANSWERS/RATIONALE

It is important to note the region(s) in which a patient describes their abdominal pain. This gives a clue to the affected organ that may be causing the pain.

The nine regions, superiorly to inferiorly and right to left, are (see Figure 12.2):

1. Right hypochondriac region—organs here include the liver, gallbladder, right kidney, right hepatic flexure of the colon, and the small intestine

2. Epigastric region—organs here include the liver, stomach, adrenal glands, the head and body of the pancreas, and part of the small intestine (duodenum)

3. Left hypochondriac region—organs here include the left tip of the liver, the stomach, the tail of the pancreas, left kidney, spleen, splenic flexure of the colon, and small intestine

4. Right lumbar region—organs here include the ascending colon, the small intestine, and the right kidney

5. Umbilical region—organs here include parts of the small intestine (duodenum and jejunum) and the transverse colon

6. Left lumbar region—organs here include the descending colon, small intestine, and the left kidney

7. Right iliac region—organs here include the appendix, cecum, inferior portion of the ascending colon, and the small intestine

8. Hypogastric region—organs here include the bladder, sigmoid colon, reproductive organs, and the small intestine

9. Left iliac region—organs here include the sigmoid colon, descending colon, and the small intestine

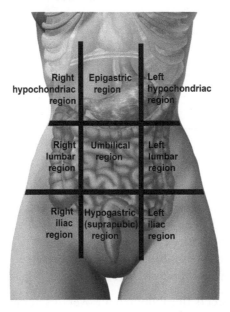

FIGURE 12.2 The nine regions of the abdomen.

QUESTION 12.3 **(Multiple response)**

Which of the following subjective information collected during the health history would be considered a risk factor for the development of liver disease? *(Select all that apply)*

A) Drinking an average of six beers a day

B) Poorly controlled diabetes

C) Poorly controlled cholesterol levels

D) Obesity

E) Cystic fibrosis

F) Hepatitis B virus

G) Heart disease

Answer: A, B, C, D, E, F, G

RATIONALE

Major modifiable risk factors for liver disease, such as cirrhosis, include heavy alcohol consumption, obesity, and high cholesterol. Unmodifiable risk factors include chronic infection with hepatitis B, C, or D; diabetes mellitus; genetic diseases, such as cystic fibrosis; and heart disease.

QUESTION 12.4 (Fill in the blank)

List the order in which physical examination of the abdomen should occur:

1. _____

2. _____

3. _____

4. _____

ANSWER(S)/RATIONALE

When performing a physical assessment of the abdomen, the patient should first be asked to lie in a supine position, with arms resting to either side of the body. This position prevents tightening of the abdominal muscles (Ignatavicius & Workman, 2016). A thorough assessment of the abdomen includes inspection, auscultation, percussion, and palpation.

The nurse first **inspects** the abdomen for overall symmetry/asymmetry and presence of discoloration, abdominal distention, and pulsations.

Next, the nurse **auscultates** all four quadrants of the abdomen with the diaphragm of a stethoscope. This should always be done prior to percussion or palpation, as the latter two assessment techniques may alter sounds (Hinkle & Cheever, 2018). The characterization of bowel sounds should be noted as normal, hypoactive, hyperactive, or absent (see Table 12.2). Bruits may be auscultated with the bell of a stethoscope. A bruit heard over the aorta may indicate the presence of an aortic aneurysm.

The nurse next **percusses** the abdomen to estimate the size of solid organs, such as the liver or spleen, and to determine the presence of fluid, air, and masses. Unless a bruit is heard, all four quadrants should be percussed and the character of sound documented (see Table 12.3; Jarvis, 2012).

Lastly, the nurse **palpates** the abdomen using light palpation to assess for tenderness and deep palpation to assess for masses (Jarvis, 2012).

TABLE 12.2 Bowel Sounds

Bowel Sound	Qualities	Possible Causes
Normal	Relatively high-pitched and irregular 5–35 sounds occurring every minute or one sound every 5–15 seconds	Normally functioning intestines
Hypoactive	Softer and widespread sounds Less than 5 sounds per minute or one occurring every 20 to 30 seconds or longer	Postoperative after general anesthesia Paralytic ileus Peritonitis Decreased bowel motility Late intestinal obstruction
Absent	Absence of intestinal motility No sounds heard for 5 minutes	Peritonitis Paralytic ileus (late finding) Perforation Mesenteric ischemia
Hyperactive	Loud and frequent, with 35 or more sounds per minute	Diarrhea Peritonitis Intestinal obstruction (early finding) Gastroenteritis Anxiety
Bruit	"Whooshing" sound over the abdominal aorta, renal arteries, and/or iliac arteries	Abdominal aortic aneurysm Renal artery stenosis

(Jarvis, 2012)

TABLE 12.3 Percussion Sounds

Sound	Intensity	Pitch	Quality	Duration	Common Locations
Resonance	Moderately loud	Low	Clear, hollow	Moderate	Over normal lung tissue
Hyper-resonance	Very loud	Very low	Booming	Long	Emphysematous lung
Tympany	Loud	High	Musical and drum-like	Longest	Enclosed air-filled space (e.g., stomach, intestines, puffed-out cheek)
Dullness	Soft	High	Muffled thud	Short	Dense organ (e.g., liver or spleen)
Flatness	Soft	High	Flat, absolute dullness	Very short	Areas with no air present (e.g., muscle, bone)

QUESTION 12.5 (Multiple choice)

The term for yellowing of skin is:

A) Jaundice

B) Icterus

C) Asterixis

D) A and B

Answer: D

RATIONALE

Jaundice and *icterus* are synonymous, and both are terms used for yellowing of skin. Jaundice may occur when there is damage to the liver, causing an inability to effectively excrete bilirubin, a byproduct of the breakdown of old red blood cells. Jaundice may also occur if there is an obstruction in the bile ducts due to scarring, edema, fibrosis, or cancer, leading to an inability to effectively excrete bilirubin (Cleveland Clinic, 2018).

Asterixis is the term used to describe a flapping tremor in the hands, particularly when the wrists are extended. Asterixis may be a sign of hepatic encephalopathy, but it can also be associated with other diseases (Zackria & John, 2023).

QUESTION 12.6 (Multiple choice)

Percussion of the sixth or seventh right intercostal space at the mid-clavicular line should yield what sound?

A) Resonance

B) Hyper-resonance

C) Dullness

D) Tympany

Answer: C

RATIONALE

The liver is located in the right upper quadrant of the abdomen (see Figure 12.3 for a view of the gastrointestinal organs), beginning at around the fifth intercostal space at the mid-clavicular line. Percussion over a dense organ would yield a dull sound.

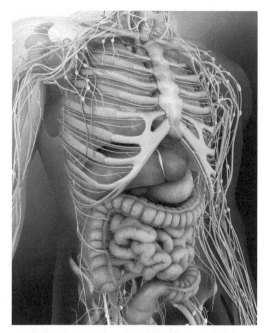

FIGURE 12.3 View of the gastrointestinal organs in relation to the skeleton.

QUESTION 12.7 (Multiple choice)

As the nurse, you would like to perform a full abdominal assessment, including an assessment for ascites. How is this performed?

A) Deep palpation at the umbilicus and at the abdominal flanks

B) Percussion of the abdomen to assess for areas of tympany and dullness

C) Auscultation for a fluid wave

D) Inspection of the abdomen for a fluid wave

Answer: B

RATIONALE

Ascites is free fluid in the peritoneal cavity; it may develop as a result of several disease processes, including heart failure, renal failure, cancer, portal hypertension, and hepatic cirrhosis. The presence of bulging flanks during inspection of the abdomen may suggest the presence of ascites. It is important to note that an obese abdomen may also have flanks that bulge (see Figure 12.4; University of Washington Department of Medicine, n.d.).

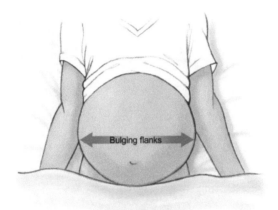

FIGURE 12.4 Bulging flanks (Liou & Price, 2021).

Percussion of the abdomen may be performed to assess areas of tympany and dullness. Starting at the umbilicus, percuss laterally to the flanks and inferiorly. The point of transition from tympany to dullness should be noted. Approximately 1,500 ml of fluid must be present in the peritoneal cavity for flank dullness to be appreciated on physical examination. If ascites is present, the fluid will shift when the patient is placed in a lateral decubitus position. Again, percussion is used to note the transition from tympany to dullness (see Figure 12.5; Liou & Price, 2021).

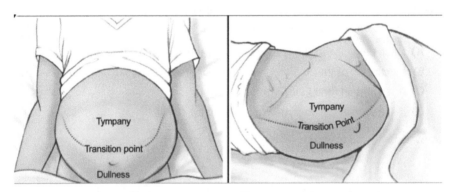

FIGURE 12.5 Assessing for flank dullness, with the patient lying supine, and shifting dullness, with the patient lying in the lateral decubitus position (Liou & Price, 2021).

Patient information continued... A CT scan of the abdomen and hepatic function tests were drawn to determine the cause of Mrs. Johnson's symptoms. The CT scan shows a nodular liver consistent with cirrhosis. Her serum bilirubin, AST, and ALT were all elevated. She is admitted to the step-down unit for further evaluation. Several hours after admission, Mrs. Johnson reports having a black, tarry, and foul-smelling stool.

QUESTION 12.8 (Multiple choice)

What is the term for black, tarry stool?

A) Hematemesis

B) Steatorrhea

C) Hematochezia

D) Melena

Answer: D

RATIONALE

Melena is the term for stool that is black with a tarry consistency. This usually indicates excessive blood accumulation in the stomach for at least 14 hours (Nettina, 2019). Sources of bleeding that may result in melena include the esophagus, stomach, and the duodenum.

Evidence of gastrointestinal bleeding is delineated in Table 12.4.

TABLE 12.4 Terminology to Describe Gastrointestinal Bleeding

GI Bleeding Term	Description
Melena	Tarry, black stool
Hematochezia	Bright red, bloody stool that is typically associated with bleeding in the lower gastrointestinal tract, such as the colon, rectum, or anus. Significant bleeding from the upper gastrointestinal tract may also result in hematochezia.
Steatorrhea	Greasy or fatty, often foul-smelling stool. Steatorrhea may occur from diseases affecting the pancreas, biliary obstruction, malabsorption syndromes, and medications, among other causes.
Hematemesis	Bright red blood that is vomited from high in the esophagus.
Coffee-ground emesis	Appearance of coffee grounds. Blood that has mixed with acid from the stomach and is vomited from the esophagus, stomach, or duodenum.

(Ansari, 2023)

Patient information continued... The medical team was immediately notified of Mrs. Johnson's melena. The patient was found to have leaking esophageal varices as a result of cirrhosis. The medical team was able to act quickly to ligate the varices and control the bleeding.

QUESTION 12.9 (Fill in the blank)

In addition to esophageal varices, what are two other potential locations of varices?

1. _____

2. _____

Answer: 1. Umbilical varices; 2. Rectal varices

RATIONALE

Varices are swollen, engorged veins that are a higher risk for rupture.

Umbilical (navel) varices may be present as a result of portal hypertension due to hepatic cirrhosis and liver failure. Varices here may be visible superficially and are termed *caput medusae* due to the similar appearance to Medusa's head (see Figure 12.6).

Rectal varices may also result from collateral circulation as a result of portal hypertension.

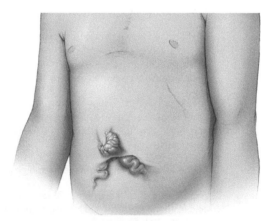

FIGURE 12.6 Caput medusae (Ramers, 2021).

QUESTION 12.10 **(Multiple response)**

In addition to the findings already discussed, what other physical findings might Mrs. Johnson have due to hepatic cirrhosis? *(Select all that apply)*

A) Bruising of the skin

B) Confusion

C) Difficulty breathing

D) Lower extremity edema

E) Fever

Answer: A, B, C, D, E

RATIONALE

The liver is a complex organ with a multitude of functions. It not only filters the blood of toxins but also synthesizes key components of coagulation, metabolism, and digestion (Johns Hopkins, n.d.).

A main function of the liver is filtration of the blood. Toxic substances, including ammonia, are converted and processed by the liver for excretion in the urine. Excessive buildup of ammonia can lead to confusion and hepatic encephalopathy. As discussed previously, the liver also breaks down old red blood cells and excretes bilirubin in bile and in urine. Excessive buildup of bilirubin can lead to jaundice (Shenvi & Serrano, 2017).

Bile produced by the liver is excreted into the small intestine to aid in the digestion of fats. Fats are then transported through the body via cholesterol, which is also produced by the liver. Another energy source used by the body, glucose, is stored in the liver in the form of glycogen. The liver converts glycogen back to glucose as needed via gluconeogenesis (Johns Hopkins, n.d.).

The liver also produces *albumin,* which is one of the most abundant proteins in the bloodstream and responsible for approximately 75% of plasma oncotic pressure (Walayat et al., 2017). A decrease in plasma albumin due to liver dysfunction coupled with portal hypertension results in third-spacing and the subsequent development of lower extremity edema and ascites. Increasing ascites may compress other internal organs, causing diminished appetite, anorexia, nausea, discomfort, and respiratory distress (Saif et al., 2009).

Many coagulation factors are produced by liver parenchymal cells. Prothrombin time and international normalized ratio can be elevated with severe liver disease. Providers may also estimate the severity of liver disease with elevated levels (Northup & Caldwell, 2013). Therefore, a patient with severe liver dysfunction may present with *purpura* (purple spots due to leaking blood vessels), *ecchymosis* (bruising), or *petechiae* (tiny brown-purple spots due to bleeding under the skin).

Lastly, the liver plays a role in the immune response, producing several molecules and factors involved in inflammation. Large populations of immune cells are also housed in the liver, phagocytizing pathogens that are brought for filtration via the portal vein. Damage to the liver, therefore, leads to a reduced ability to sense and mount a response to systemic inflammation (Robinson et al., 2016).

CHAPTER 12 WORKSHEET

Based on my initial assessment, I thought:

_____

_____

_____

Based on my revised/informed assessment, I now know:

_____

_____

_____

A nursing priority for this patient would be _____

because _____

After completing this chapter, something I have learned is:

_____

_____

_____

After completing this chapter, something I need more clarity on is:

_____

_____

_____

After completing this chapter, something else I want to learn is:

_____

_____

_____

REFERENCES

Ansari, P. (2023). Overview of gastrointestinal bleeding. *Merck Manual Professional Version*. https://www.merckmanuals.com/professional/gastrointestinal-disorders/gastrointestinal-bleeding/overview-of-gastrointestinal-bleeding?query=gastrointestinal%20bleeding

Cleveland Clinic. (n.d.). *Adult jaundice.* https://my.clevelandclinic.org/health/diseases/15367-adult-jaundice

Douglas, M. E., Randleman, M. L., DeLane, A. M., & Palmer, G. A. (2014). Determining pain scale preference in a veteran population experiencing chronic pain. *Pain Management Nursing, 15*(3), 625–631. https://doi.org/10.1016/j.pmn.2013.06.003

Hinkle, J. L., & Cheever, K. H. (2018). *Brunner and Suddarth's textbook of medical-surgical nursing, Volume 2* (14th ed.). Wolters Kluwer.

Ignatavicius, D. D., & Workman, M. L. (2016). *Medical-surgical nursing: Patient-centered collaborative care* (8th ed.). Elsevier.

Jarvis, C. (2012). *Physical examination and health assessment* (6th ed.). Saunders.

Johns Hopkins. (n.d.). *Liver: Anatomy and functions.* https://www.hopkinsmedicine.org/health/conditions-and-diseases/liver-anatomy-and-functions

Liou, I. W., & Price, J. (2021). *Diagnosis and management of ascites.* https://www.hepatitisc.uw.edu/go/management-cirrhosis-related-complications/ascites-diagnosis-management/core-concept/all#figures

Mankoski, A. (2000). *Mankoski pain scale.* http://www.valis.com/andi/painscale.html

McCaffery, M., & Beebe, A. (1989). *Pain: Clinical manual for nursing practice.* Mosby.

Nettina, S. (2019). *Lippincott manual of nursing practice* (11th ed.). Wolters Kluwer.

Northup, P. G., & Caldwell, S. H. (2013). Coagulation in liver disease: A guide for the clinician. *Clinical Gastroenterology and Hepatology, 11,* 1064–1074. https://doi.org/10.1016/j.cgh.2013.02.026

Ramers, C. B. (2021). *Initial evaluation of persons with chronic hepatitis C.* https://www.hepatitisc.uw.edu/go/evaluation-staging-monitoring/initial-evaluation-chronic/core-concept/all

Robinson, M. W., Harmon, C., & O'Farrelly, C. (2016). Liver immunology and its role in inflammation and homeostasis. *Cellular and Molecular Immunology, 13*(3), 267–276. https://doi.org/10.1038/cmi.2016.3

Saif, M. W., Siddiqui, I. A., & Sohail, M. A. (2009). Management of ascites due to gastrointestinal malignancy. *Annals of Saudi Medicine, 29*(5), 369–377.

Shenvi, C., & Serrano, K. (2017, Dec. 22). Hyperammonemia: Is it the liver or something else? *Emergency Physicians Monthly.* https://epmonthly.com/article/hyperammonemia-liver-something-else/

University of Washington Department of Medicine. (n.d.). *Techniques: Liver & ascites.* https://depts.washington.edu/physdx/liver/tech.html

Walayat, S., Martin, D., Patel, J., Ahmed, U., Asghar, M. N, Pai, A. U., & Dhillon, S. (2017). Role of albumin in cirrhosis: From a hospitalist's perspective. *Journal of Community Hospital Internal Medicine Perspectives, 7*(1), 8–14. https://doi.org/10.1080/20009666.2017.1302704

Zackria, R., & John, S. (2023). Asterixis. *StatPearls.* https://www.ncbi.nlm.nih.gov/books/NBK535445/

CHAPTER 13

Genitourinary and Sexual Health

Carrie D. Michalski, JD, MSN, RN

 CASE STUDY

Patient Presenting to Primary Care With Abdominal Pain

- 17-year-old female
- Lying on side, splinting abdomen

T 99.1°F oral	HR 88 bpm	BP 122/74	RR 16	O2 98%	Pain 6/10

Abigail, a 17-year-old female student, presents to the community center with complaints of abdominal pain. Abigail was born and reared in the United States, is of Caucasian descent, and is a nonpracticing Protestant. She lives with her parents and has health insurance through her father's work health plan. The family has received primary care from the community center facility for the past 10 years.

The patient and her mother are together in the examination room when the nurse enters. The nurse notes the mother sitting in the chair. Abigail is lying on the examination table on her right side, with her knees pulled close to her abdomen and her hands holding her lower abdomen. She has no history of gastrointestinal or abdominal issues. She also denies any food intolerances or eating anything unusual or uncharacteristic of her usual diet. She is not experiencing nausea or vomiting. She is not crying but grimacing with a creased brow.

Prior to the nurse entering, the nursing assistant reported the vital signs listed above.

QUESTION 13.1 (True or false)

"Guarding" is a term used to describe a person holding a body part in an attempt to protect or relieve pain.

    A) True   **B)** False

Answer: A

RATIONALE

Terms like guarding and splinting can be used interchangeably. The patient may use guarding or splinting to support, protect, or stabilize a body part from movement that can elicit pain (Venes, 2013). The patient may hold or support the affected body part as a protective measure when they move, or they may involuntarily tense their muscles when a provider is performing an assessment to the affected area. In the present case, the patient is using her hands to hold her lower abdomen, indicating nonverbally the area of discomfort or pain. While this behavior is a sign of nonverbal communication, the nurse will confirm what is being seen by asking specific clarifying questions and conducting a full pain assessment.

Clinical reasoning is the process of collecting information through a variety of sources to determine a diagnosis and ultimately the plan of treatment (Venes, 2013). A collection of different data points comes from what the patient and/or family says, responses to questions about symptoms, prior medical records, signs revealed during the physical examination, and laboratory results and other diagnostic imaging (e.g., ultrasound or radiology). The clinical reasoning method starts by determining through clues, both verbal and nonverbal, what could be the cause of the patient's complaint—in this case, abdominal pain.

An initial consideration is the organs located in the defined area of the abdomen and then the possible conditions that may be causing the issues. This process begins before we even speak to the patient. Just by knowing the chief complaint along with anatomy and physiology, the nurse begins the thinking process that informs their actions through collecting history, formulating the appropriate questions, and performing an assessment.

The abdominopelvic cavity is the space between the bottom edges of the rib cage and superior to the pelvic bones. This area can be divided into either four or nine different sections (Jarvis, 2020). Division of the abdomen into four quadrants is simplest, using the umbilicus as the center point. However, utilizing the nine regions can be more helpful due to the many organs and the number of possible conditions to be evaluated. See Figure 13.1 and Table 13.1.

4 Quadrants

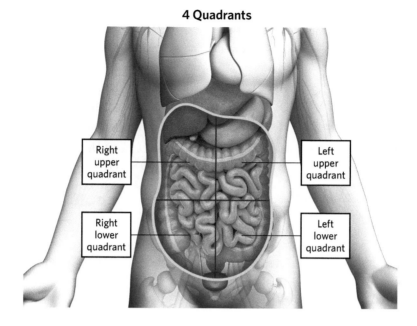

9 Regions

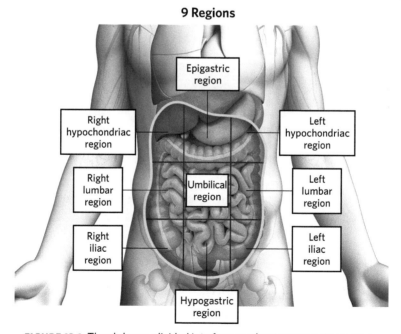

FIGURE 13.1 The abdomen divided into four quadrants versus nine regions.

QUESTION 13.2 **(Multiple response)**

Identify the organs located in the lower region of the abdominopelvic cavity: *(Select all that apply)*

A) Appendix	**F)** Liver	**K)** Spleen
B) Bladder	**G)** Pancreas	**L)** Transverse colon
C) Cecum	**H)** Rectum	**M)** Prostate
D) Gallbladder	**I)** Sigmoid colon	**N)** Uterus/ovaries
E) Kidney	**J)** Small intestine	**O)** Stomach

Answer(s): A, B, C, H, I, J, M, N

TABLE 13.1 **Nine Abdominal Regions**

Right Hypochondriac	Epigastric	Left Hypochondriac
Ascending colon	Esophagus	Descending colon
Gallbladder	Liver	Left kidney
Liver	Pancreas	Liver
Right kidney	Right and left adrenal glands	Pancreas
Small intestine	Right and left kidneys	Small intestine
Transverse colon	Small intestine	Spleen
	Spleen	Stomach
	Stomach	Transverse colon
	Transverse colon	

Right Lumbar	Umbilical	Left Lumbar
Ascending colon	Cisterna chyli	Descending colon
Gallbladder	Pancreas	Left kidney
Liver	Right and left kidneys	Small intestine
Right kidney	Right and left ureters	
Small intestine	Small intestine	
	Stomach	
	Transverse colon	

Right Iliac	Hypogastric	Left Iliac
Appendix	Prostate	Left fallopian tubes (F)
Cecum	Rectum	Left ovary (F)
Ascending colon	Right and left fallopian tubes (F)	Small intestine
Right fallopian tube (F)	Right and left ovaries (F)	Descending colon
Right ovary (F)	Right and left ureters	Sigmoid colon
Small intestine	Seminal vesicle (M)	
	Sigmoid colon	
	Small intestine	
	Urinary bladder	
	Uterus (F)	
	Vas deferens (M)	

(Study.com, n.d.)

QUESTION 13.3 (Multiple response)

Based on the location of those specific organs, identify the possible conditions that could be the cause of the chief complaint—acute pain in the lower hypogastric or suprapubic region. Select from the list: *(Select all that apply)*

A) Cholecystitis

B) Peptic ulcer

C) Menstrual-related conditions

D) Pregnancy

E) Sexually transmitted infection (STI)

F) Pelvic inflammatory disease

G) Endometriosis

H) Constipation

I) GERD

J) Cirrhosis of the liver

K) Ovarian cysts

L) Appendicitis

M) Splenomegaly

N) Pancreatitis

O) Cystitis/urinary tract infection (UTI)

Answer(s): C, D, E, F, G, H, K, L, O

RATIONALE

Utilizing Table 13.1, the female organs in the lower hypogastric or suprapubic region include the uterus with its connecting fallopian tubes and ovaries as well as the genitourinary (bladder) and gastrointestinal organs. The lower quadrants house the large and small intestines, the cecum, the appendix, and the sigmoid colon and rectum. Answers C through G and K relate to the female reproductive organs. Answer H is associated with the lower large intestines on the left iliac and hypogratric regions. Answer L—appendicitis—would be a result of pain stemming from the appendix, located on the right iliac region. Answer O relates to the bladder. Cystitis is an inflammation or infection in the bladder, whereas a UTI can include other parts of the urinary tract.

QUESTION 13.4 (Multiple choice)

After introductions, the nurse begins to ask questions about the patient's pain symptoms. Which question speaks to the quality of the pain?

A) "Would you please point to the pain?"

B) "Would you please describe the pain?"

C) "When did the pain start?"

D) "Please rate your pain on a scale from 0–10, with zero being no pain and 10 being the worst imaginable pain."

Answer: B

RATIONALE

Exploration of the chief complaint can be done in a systematic manner utilizing the mnemonic PQRST (Jarvis, 2020) or OLD CARTS (Thompson, 2018; see Figure 13.2). These tools help lead the interviewer so they may understand the patient's pain experience. These mnemonics identify specific questions to analyze the patient's pain and will help to elicit accurate and clear information. Regardless of the mnemonic used, the questions are similar.

PQRST	**OLD CARTS**
• **P:** Provocation/Palliation Factors: What makes the pain better? Worse?	• **O:** Onset: When did it start?
• **Q:** Quality: Describe the pain?	• **L:** Location: Where is it located?
• **R:** Region/Radiation: Can you point to where it hurts? Does the pain move?	• **D:** Duration: How long has this gone on/how long does it last? Is it constant, or does it come and go?
• **S:** Severity/Scale: Pain scale 0-10	• **C:** Characteristics: How does it feel?
• **T:** Timing: Is the pain constant or intermittent? How long have you had this pain?	• **A:** Aggravating/Alleviating Factors: What makes it worse? What makes it better?
	• **R:** Relieving Factors: What makes it better?
	• **T:** Treatment: How do you relieve the pain?
	• **S:** Severity/Scale: Pain scale 0-10

FIGURE 13.2 PQRST vs. OLD CARTS.

Patient information continued... In response to the health history and PQRST questions, Abigail describes the following:

PQRST Category	Patient Statement	Further Nursing Assessment
Provocation/ Palliation Factor	"Going to the bathroom makes it worse. But I have to keep going to the bathroom."	Voiding makes it worse. Patient also describes urinary frequency without significant results. Patient had a bowel movement yesterday and typically defecates once daily. That bowel movement was brown and passed easily; she did not experience diarrhea or constipation.
Quality	"When I go to the bathroom, I feel more pressure when I pee, and it burns. And I feel pain and pressure constantly now."	Patient states her urine is darker than normal.

PQRST Category	Patient Statement	Further Nursing Assessment
Region/ Radiation	"It doesn't move; it constantly hurts here, and it is getting worse."	Patient indicates her lower, center, hypogastric, or suprapubic region.
Severity/Scale	"It is a 6 out of 10. I have never felt anything like this. It hurts so much!"	Patient grimaces and holds her lower abdomen.
Timing	"It started yesterday afternoon; it is constant pressure and getting worse."	Patient states she feels monthly menstrual cramps occasionally, but what she feels now is different from menstrual cramps.

QUESTION 13.5 (Multiple choice)

When assessing a teenage patient in the presence of a parent or caregiver, the nurse is mindful of all the following except:

A) Explaining expectations of the interaction

B) Asking permission to discuss sensitive topics in the presence of the parent/caregiver

C) Providing adequate privacy

D) Demanding the parent/caregiver leave the room for the exam

Answer: D

RATIONALE

To be mindful of the patient's experience, it is important to provide privacy and explain expectations, as well as ask permission to discuss these more sensitive topics (Santa Maria et al., 2017).

In the current scenario, remember that the mother of this teenager is also in the room. It is necessary to ensure that the patient is comfortable responding to the next set of questions in the presence of others. Also recognize that the integrity of the information may be compromised if gathering information with the adolescent's parent in the room. Even if the patient is truthful, it can create an awkward or embarrassing atmosphere for the patient to be discussing sexual behaviors and experiences in front of a parent (Fuzzell et al., 2016; Nemours TeensHealth, n.d.; Santa Maria et al., 2017).

It is best to begin with a statement that all female patients are asked questions about their menstrual history and sexual health. The conversation about menstrual history is generally less of a sensitive issue and is therefore a good starting point (KidsHealth, 2018). To begin, it might be easier to discuss when they started their menses, when they had their last menstrual period (LMP), and information about their menstrual cycle (regularity, blood loss, pain, energy level, physical and emotional symptoms), then lead into questions about their sexual history and health.

Patient information continued... When exploring menstrual history, the patient states: menarche at 14 years old, LMP two months ago (assist the patient to provide an actual date). Cycle 28–32 days, lasts 4–5 days, irregular pattern, "may miss a month." Over the last year her periods have become more regular. Most months the patient does not experience menstrual cramping. Blood loss is described as a day of spotting at the beginning and at the end, with two to three days of moderate bleeding. Occasionally she will experience one heavy day.

QUESTION 13.6 (Multiple choice)

Which of the following statements by the nurse is most appropriate to address the patient's right to privacy and to be respectful of the patient's choice?

A) "Since you brought your mother with you to the appointment, I will assume you want her present during the history and exam."

B) "I like to talk to my teen patients alone so they can start taking a role in their healthcare and be comfortable asking any questions."

C) "Abigail, if you want your mother to leave the room, you will have to ask her."

D) "Mom, I am going to have to ask you to leave the room so that your daughter has privacy and will feel free to ask questions."

Answer: B

RATIONALE

Patients have a right to privacy, but they also have a right to decide who will be with them in the examination room. If it is the patient's choice to be alone with the provider, the provider can advocate for the patient's privacy. Providing the desired environment will promote a healthy therapeutic relationship and encourage more accurate, honest conversation (Santa Maria et al., 2017). Confidentiality may be an unfamiliar topic for the adolescent. Explaining to adolescents that they have the freedom to share information and concerns in private without the parent being told is a good directive to begin the conversation (Fuzzell et al., 2016).

At this point we have an acute situation—pain in the lower hypogastric region. This is the nursing priority and needs to be the focus right now. However, the patient should be encouraged to make a follow-up appointment with added attention to other sexual health issues (American College of Obstetricians and Gynecologists [ACOG], 2022).

There is a distinction between obtaining a sexual history and sexual health. A more thorough conversation with this patient about sexual health is warranted once revealed she is in a sexual relationship without consistent birth control or gynecological care. Sexual health is a broader discussion about sexuality and its connection to physical health. It would include sexual satisfaction, sexual identity, prevention of undesired pregnancy, sexually transmitted disease, pelvic pain, as well as other factors (Kinsburg, 2006).

However, the current priority is to determine whether the chief complaint is related to uterine issues, specific to menstrual- and/or pregnancy-related conditions. Some focused, specific questions might include:

- Are you sexually active?
- Do you engage in sex with females, males, or both?
- Are you presently in a relationship that involves sexual intercourse?
- Do you use any forms of birth control?
- Do you experience dyspareunia (difficult or painful intercourse)?
- Have you ever been pregnant?
- How many sexual partners have you had?
- Do you know if any of your sexual partners have had an STI or STD?
- Have you received gynecological care?

Patient information continued... Abigail states that she has a boyfriend, also 17 years old. They go to school together and have been dating for almost 10 months. They have been experimenting with oral sex over the past six months. They have had vaginal intercourse six times in the last two to three months using coitus interruptus (withdrawal). They did use a condom the last time they had sexual intercourse, which was two days ago.

The patient further states this is the only boy with whom she has done more than just kissing. She believes her boyfriend was also a virgin when they began their relationship. She has never been pregnant and has never received gynecological care.

QUESTION 13.7 **(Fill in the blank)**

Critically think through the collected data, and list any concerning clinical assessment data:

1. _____

2. _____

3. _____

4. _____

5. _____

6. _____

7. _____

 ANSWERS/RATIONALE

1. Vital signs: low-grade fever, potentially signaling an infection, not necessarily indicating the location of the infection.

2. Pain in the lower hypogastric region: potentially a problem with the female reproductive system, the genitourinary system, and/or a gastrointestinal condition.

3. Urinary urgency and frequency without results: potentially indicative of a UTI and/or pregnancy. While frequent urination could be either condition, the qualifier of frequency "without results" is more in line with a UTI.

4. Burning with urination, another classic sign potentially indicative of a UTI.

5. Onset of pain two days ago, after intercourse, which is getting worse: the fact that the pain is increasing in intensity, not going away, and after intercourse is notable for an association with UTI.

6. Sexual intercourse without protection: While no birth control protection is 100% effective, the fact that no protection was used during intercourse introduces a real possibility of pregnancy.

7. LMP (actual date) two months ago with a past history of irregular periods: Even if a menstrual cycle is irregular, ovulation can still occur; therefore, a person can still get pregnant. A history of irregular periods complicates the process of identifying whether menstruation is late, which can delay getting early reproductive care.

QUESTION 13.8 (Fill in the blank)

List the two system assessments that will be the focus of the physical examination.

1. _____

2. _____

ANSWER/RATIONALE

The two systems that will be the focus of the physical examination are assessment of the genitourinary system and assessment of the female reproductive system.

The focused assessment of the urinary system includes the urethra, bladder, ureters, and kidney (see Figure 13.3). Bacteria can enter the urethra and progress into the bladder. Particularly due to the short urethra in the female anatomy, women have a higher incidence of UTI risk (ACOG, 2024; Mishra et al., 2018). Another name for a bladder infection is cystitis.

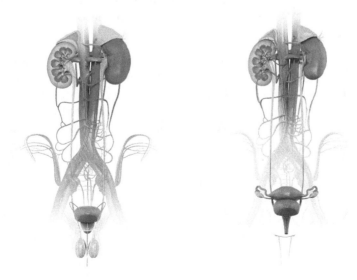

FIGURE 13.3 Human urinary systems.

QUESTION 13.9 (Multiple choice)

When evaluating for potential inflammation of the kidney, the nurse utilizes which assessment technique?

A) CVA tenderness

B) Rebound tenderness

C) Murphy's sign

D) Bowel sounds

Answer: A

RATIONALE

If the bacteria continue to invade, it can advance into the ureter and affect the kidney. Pyelonephritis is another term for a kidney infection. An upper urinary infection, involving the ureters and kidneys, can be more serious than in the lower urinary system. To assess the kidneys for signs of infection, perform costovertebral angle (CVA) tenderness. Kidney tenderness may be indicative of inflammation. In addition to pain, other symptoms of pyelonephritis are fever, chills, nausea, and bloody or odorous urine (ACOG, 2024; Matuszkiewicz-Rowińska et al., 2015; Mishra et al., 2018).

Assist the patient to a seated position and place your nondominant hand on the patient's back at the level of the twelfth thoracic vertebrae (T-12). A portion of your hand will be on and below the posterior ribs on either side of the spine (see Figure 13.4). In the case of pyelonephritis, this touch alone may produce tenderness. If that is the case, then the exam stops and the documentation will state: "positive CVA tenderness with palpation." If the patient is not uncomfortable with palpation, then an indirect percussion method is used to assess for CVA tenderness (Jarvis, 2020; Thompson, 2018).

To perform percussion for CVA tenderness, place one palm at T-12, percuss using a fisted hand, and thud the ulnar edge onto the dorsal side of the hand positioned at T-12 (Jarvis, 2020). If the first thud did not elicit a tenderness response, then repeat the strike a little more forcefully. If either the first or second strike yields tenderness, then again the documentation would read: "positive CVA tenderness with indirect percussion." Another expression for CVA tenderness is flank pain. It is possible to have CVA tenderness in one or both sides, and the location of tenderness should be documented accordingly.

Costovertebral Angle Tenderness

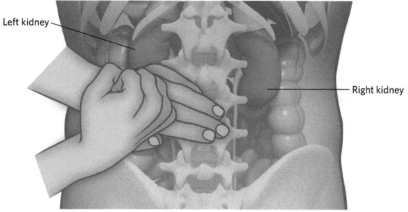

Left kidney

Right kidney

FIGURE 13.4 Percussion to assess for CVA tenderness.

Prior to positioning the patient for the gynecological exam, it is considerate to offer the patient bathroom access. This particular patient in our case study does not need encouragement because she is experiencing urgency to void. But all patients would be more comfortable given the opportunity to empty their bladder prior to the external and internal gynecological assessment (Jarvis, 2020). Additionally, obtaining a urine sample also has benefits for our case study patient's concerns.

Patient information continued... In consultation with the provider, the nurse obtains the following orders:

- Mid-stream urine specimen for urine analysis
- Urine culture and sensitivity sample
- Pregnancy test

Once the orders are received, the nurse's initial action is to assess the patient by two identifiers and to ensure the patient is aware of the purpose of the orders. Since the patient will be performing the clean catch in private, it is also necessary to confirm that the patient understands the method of collection. Therefore, the nurse performs patient education on the steps to obtain a clean-void or mid-stream specimen. After the nurse explains the items in the kit and reviews the steps, it is best practice to provide a visual step-by-step illustration for improved compliance (Eley et al., 2016)

QUESTION 13.10 (Sequencing)

Place the following steps in the correct order to obtaining a clean mid-stream urine specimen.

A) Close container without touching the inside of the container or the lid.

B) Still holding the labia, initiate a stream of urine.

C) Clean external container before handing it to the nurse, then perform hand hygiene.

D) Spread the labia with one hand.

E) The patient should perform hand hygiene.

F) Wipe using a front-to-back technique (urethral opening toward anus) with three strokes using the provided wipes. One wipe for each stroke: first on the further side, the closest side, and then down the middle.

G) Remove container before ending stream of urine or releasing labia and complete voiding.

H) Pass container into urine flow and collect urine.

I) Prepare the sterile supplies without touching the inside of the container or lid.

Answer: E, I, D, F, B, H, G, A, C

 RATIONALE

The steps to obtaining a mid-stream urine sample, in the correct order, are:

1. The patient should perform hand hygiene.
2. Prepare the sterile supplies without touching the inside of the container or lid.
3. Spread the labia with one hand.
4. Wipe using a front-to-back technique (urethral opening toward anus) with three strokes using the provided wipes. One wipe for each stroke: first on the further side, the closest side, and then down the middle.
5. Still holding the labia, initiate a stream of urine.
6. Pass container into urine flow and collect urine.
7. Remove container before ending stream of urine or releasing labia and complete voiding.
8. Close container without touching the inside of the container or the lid.
9. Clean external container before handing it to the nurse, then perform hand hygiene.

(Lough et al., 2019; Potter et al., 2017)

When the patient has completed collection of urine, the nurse will don gloves and take the container. The nurse will assess the urine for color, clarity, odor, and amount. The nurse may, using proper agency protocol, also collect urine for other tests as ordered. Thereafter, the nurse will affix proper patient identification labels and place in a specimen bag as required by their agency and send to the laboratory. Upon completion of the orders, the nurse will remove gloves and perform hand hygiene.

The culture and sensitivity results will take a few days, but the urinalysis laboratory results will be ready within hours (ACOG, 2024). A quick urine analysis can be performed with a urine dip using a chemical strip. The urine pregnancy test can also be performed in the moment with quick results.

> *Patient information continued...* The patient did not experience CVA tenderness. The urine characteristics were concentrated and cloudy, yellow in color. The urine dip revealed positive for microscopic hematuria and leukocytes in the urine, and the pregnancy test was positive. The patient's obstetrical status is G1P0.

QUESTION 13.11 (Multiple choice)

What is the correct term to describe a female pregnant for the first time?

A) Primigravada   **B)** Nulliparous   **C)** Antenatal   **D)** Postpartum

Answer: A

RATIONALE

A person pregnant for the first time is considered a primigravada. Other terminology is also used to document and summarize the patient's obstetrical status. The initials G (gravida) and P (para or parity) are common documentation abbreviations. The initial "G" stands for the number of pregnancies regardless of outcome, and "P" stands for the number of pregnancies reaching 20 weeks gestation at birth regardless of fetal status at birth (White, 2018). Gravida and para are focused on the pregnancies or mother's perspective. Further abbreviations can be documented to shift the perspective to consider the fetal outcomes. In this instance, GTPAL is used:

- **G**—Gravida
- **T**—Term deliveries, after 37 weeks gestation
- **P**—Preterm deliveries, 20–37 weeks gestation
- **A**—Abortions < 20 weeks gestation (including miscarriages and therapeutic or voluntary terminations)
- **L**—Number of living children

QUESTION 13.12 **(Fill in the blank)**

Nagel's rule is a common and effective method of establishing the estimated day of birth (EDB). To use this method, start with the first day of the LMP. Then subtract three months and add seven days plus one year (White, 2018). An alternative is to add seven days and count forward nine months. Calculate the EDB based on the following LMP:

1. September 13, 2023 _____

2. December 1, 2023 _____

3. January 27, 2024 _____

4. July 16, 2024 _____

 ANSWER/RATIONALE

1. June 20, 2024

   Calculation: September 2023 – 3 months = June 2023
   13 + 7 days = 20
   next year 2024

2. September 8, 2024

   Calculation: December 2023 – 3 months = September 2023
   1 + 7 days = 8
   next year 2024

3. November 3, 2024

   Calculation: January 2024 – 3 months = October 2023
   27 + 7 days = 34 (but 31 days in October = November 3)
   next year 2024

4. April 23, 2025

   Calculation: July 2024 – 3 months = April 2024
   16 + 7 days = 23
   next year 2025

QUESTION 13.13 (Matching)

Match the female genitalia nomenclature (see Figure 13.5) with the definition of the structure:

Genitalia Structure	Definition
1. Perineum	a. The folds of skin on either side of the vaginal opening. They are the lateral borders of the vulva. There are two sets, the majora (outside) and the minora (internal).
2. Introitus	b. A small, pea-shaped, erectile structure located below the mons pubis at the top of the vulva. It is highly sensitive to tactile stimulation.
3. Os	c. The area between the vaginal opening and the anus
4. Vulva	d. Mouth or opening of the cervix
5. Urethra meatus	e. The external female genitalia from the mons pubis to the anus
6. Uterus	f. A dimple appearance, posterior to the clitoris
7. Clitoris	g. The opening entrance to the vagina
8. Vagina	h. A pear-shaped, thick-walled, muscular organ
9. Ovaries	i. One of two almond-shaped glands responsible for releasing hormones relative to the menstrual cycle
10. Labia	j. The passageway between the vulva and the cervix

(Venes, 2013; White, 2018)

Answers: 1. c; 2. g; 3. d; 4. e; 5. f; 6. h; 7. b; 8. j; 9. i; 10. a

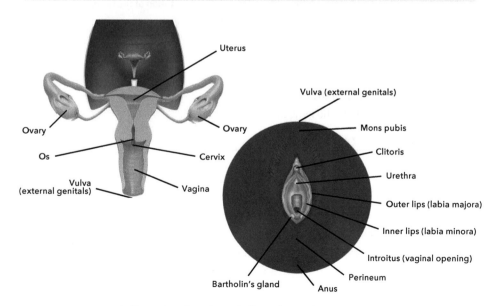

FIGURE 13.5 Female genitalia and reproductive organs.

RATIONALE

Each term above has only one appropriate definition.

The external and internal female genitalia undergo changes related to pregnancy. Externally, the labia may appear full as a result of the hormones of pregnancy. Upon internal examination of a pregnant woman, there are three specific changes to assess:

1. Chadwick's sign
2. Goodell's sign
3. Heger's sign

Sign	Clinical Characteristics
Chadwick's sign	Apparent after the first six to eight weeks. Viewed during a speculum examination, the vaginal wall and cervix can take on a bluish tinge or purple hue as a result of increased vascularity and engorgement (White, 2018).
Goodell's sign	Assessed during palpation of the cervix.
	This is a softening of the cervix related to the increase of the hormones estrogen and progesterone.
	In the nonpregnant state, the cervix is firm to palpation. In pregnancy, the cervix becomes softer and more pliable (Jarvis, 2020).
Heger's sign	Hegar's sign can be recognized while performing a bimanual examination and refers to softening of both the cervix and the uterine isthmus, creating a forward rotation of the uterus.
	Hegar's sign will also be noted early in the pregnancy between weeks 4 to 6 of gestation (Jarvis, 2020).

QUESTION 13.14 (Fill in the blank)

Name the three parts to the gynecological examination:

1. _____

2. _____

3. _____

Answers: 1. External examination; 2. Speculum examination; 3. Bimanual pelvic examination

RATIONALE

External examination is inspection and palpation of the external genitalia, assessing the vulva. Speculum examination is the inspection and palpation of the internal genitalia, using an instrument called a speculum to open the walls of the vagina for inspection and specimen collection (see Figure 13.6). In a bimanual pelvic examination, two hands are used to simultaneously assess the internal and external reproductive organs. Internally, one or two lubricated fingers of one gloved hand perform an examination palpating the vagina and cervix. The other hand is on the lower abdomen palpating the uterus and other reproductive organs from an external position. The two hands work in unison to assess size, features, location, and position relative to the other organs (Eley et al., 2016).

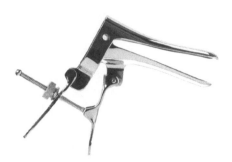

FIGURE 13.6 Speculum.

Preparation for the female gynecological physical exam includes collecting the equipment and positioning and draping the patient. A nurse being familiar with the process is a benefit to the patient. Through patient education, the nurse can share expectations of the exam to reassure the patient and make her more comfortable.

The nurse should be aware of the different sizes and types of speculums. Speculums come in both disposable plastic and metal. A patient may be unprepared for the clicking sound that is made when the speculum is opened, so informing them beforehand can calm them (Nemours TeensHealth, n.d.).

The lithotomy position is typically used for the gynecological examination (see Figure 13.7). The patient is undressed from the waist down and draped. The patient is supine, with their knees apart and feet in the stirrups. It is advisable to have the patient keep their socks on because the metal stirrups can be cold. Adjustments of the stirrup can make the patient more comfortable. Recognize that this position can make the patient feel especially vulnerable and/or embarrassed, particularly if the patient has a history of trauma, a past negative experience, or is currently in pain or in an emotional state. Communicating through the examination, offering a hand to hold, sharing information, and informing of expectations are all techniques to help the patient relax during the examination (Nemours TeensHealth, n.d.; Urology Care Foundation, 2019).

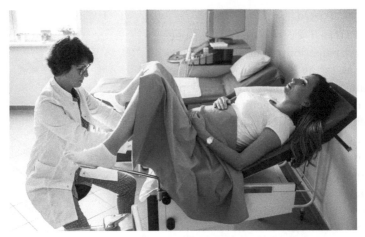

FIGURE 13.7 The lithotomy position.

The complete female reproductive system examination is usually only performed by specially trained nurses or a physician. The sequence of inspection and palpation of the external genitalia is performed first, followed by internal inspection and palpation. The generalist nurse may combine assessment of the external genitalia with patient bathing, toileting, or medication administration.

Inspect the appearance of the vulva as appropriate for the stated sex and assess for expected findings: urethral and vaginal openings, clitoris and labia structure, perineum, anus for hemorrhoids (Thompson & Scannell, 2018). Continue inspecting the skin color and condition, hair pattern, discharge, odor, swelling, bruising, rashes, piercings, lesions, lice, scars, fissures, and varicosities.

Palpate the vagina with a gloved hand for tenderness, swelling, and discharge. Particularly note the locations of 4 o'clock and 8 o'clock at the position of the Bartholin's glands and at the 1 o'clock and 11 o'clock locations for the Skene's glands (Thompson & Scannell, 2018). There should not be any inflammation or redness in these areas, which could indicate an infection or blockage.

Even though it is not the common role of the generalist nurse to perform an examination of the female internal genitalia, the nurse should be knowledgeable about the process to assist the provider and for patient teaching and expectations. Assisting with the internal genitalia examination may involve obtaining and/or holding the speculum or adjusting the light to visualize the cervix and obtain specimens. It is not unusual for the patient to feel a brief pinch or twinge when specimens are being collected.

The cervix should be assessed for color, position, size, condition of the os, surface of the cervix, and presence of secretions. The cervix should be smooth, firm, rounded, and mobile. The uterus and adnexa should not be enlarged, tender, fixed, or nodular. The ovaries are often not palpable, but if they are, they should be small, movable, oval, and smooth (Jarvis, 2020).

Patient information continued… Speculum examination revealed positive Chadwick's sign. Specimens collected for STI—gonorrhea and chlamydia, and a pap test. Bimanual examination revealed a slightly enlarged uterus at approximately the size of an avocado, 7–8 cm, consistent with an eight-week gestation pregnancy. Discussion with the patient revealed she "thinks she wants to keep the pregnancy." Referral was made to the obstetrical service for an intake pregnancy appointment and obstetrical ultrasound. Antibiotics were prescribed for the UTI, as well as prenatal vitamins. Discharge teaching was ordered.

QUESTION 13.15 (Fill in the blank)

The nurse is providing patient education. Based on the case study information and the diagnosis of UTI and early pregnancy, what are the educational priorities for our case study patient upon discharge?

1. _____

2. _____

3. _____

4. _____

 ANSWER(S)/RATIONALE

The educational priorities for the case study patient include:

1. Medication orders and instructions
2. Understanding risks and recognizing signs & symptoms of UTI
3. Prevention of UTI
4. Referral for OB/GYN care and expectations of the intake obstetrical appointment

The nurse will ask the patient about their history of allergies and the pharmacy location so the prescription can be called to a pharmacy of convenience for the patient. The medication should be taken as directed, and even if the patient's condition improves, she should take the medication until it is finished. The expected prescriptions included an antibiotic to treat the UTI and prenatal vitamins.

Understanding the risks for UTI and the signs and symptoms is needed to prevent and treat the infection early before the bacteria has had the opportunity to advance higher into the upper urinary tract. Incidence is higher in women than men, particularly those who are sexually active. Incidence is higher after engaging in sexual intercourse. Due to elevated sugar levels, diabetics are at higher risk of developing a UTI. Pregnancy can also increase the possibility of UTI. Symptoms of UTI can include painful and frequent urination described as burning, whereas more severe symptoms of fever, nausea, vomiting, and flank pain can indicate pyelonephritis. There are simple tips for preventing UTIs (Mishra et al., 2018; Urology Care Foundation, 2019):

- Stay hydrated with water.
- Urinate with urge; don't try to hold it instead of relieving your bladder.
- Clean the genital area, particularly after voiding or having a bowel movement. It is important to wipe from front (below the mons pubis) to back (anus) when using the bathroom.
- Empty the bladder before and after sex.

Briefly explain the importance of early and regular pregnancy care. Because the vaginal examination was already performed and the specimens were obtained, it will not be necessary to complete another gynecological exam at her first intake appointment. Generally, the vaginal exam won't happen again until a few weeks before expected delivery unless there is a medically indicated reason. However, the patient can expect an obstetrical ultrasound to assess the fetal heartbeat and location, baseline blood work, and pregnancy teaching. It is very likely the OB/GYN provider will follow up with another urine culture within one to two weeks after treatment (Matuszkiewicz-Rowińska et al., 2015).

CHAPTER 13 WORKSHEET

Based on my initial assessment, I thought:

_____

_____

_____

Based on my revised/informed assessment, I now know:

_____

_____

_____

A nursing priority for this patient would be _____

because _____

After completing this chapter, something I have learned is:

_____

_____

_____

After completing this chapter, something I need more clarity on is:

_____

_____

_____

After completing this chapter, something else I want to learn is:

_____

_____

_____

REFERENCES

American College of Obstetricians and Gynecologists. (2022). *Your first gynecologic visit (especially for teens).* https://www.acog.org/store/products/patient-education/pamphlets/especially-for-teens/your-first-gynecologic-visit

American College of Obstetricians and Gynecologists. (2024, January). *Urinary tract infections (UTIs).* https://www.acog.org/womens-health/faqs/urinary-tract-infections

Eley, R., Judge, C., Knight, L., Dimeski, G., & Sinnott. M. (2016). Illustrations reduce contamination of midstream urine samples in the emergency department. *Journal of Clinical Pathology, 69*(10), 921–925. https://doi.org/10.1136/jclinpath-2015-203504

Fuzzell, L., Fedesco, H. N., Alexander, S. C., Fortenberry, J. D., & Shields, C. G. (2016). "I just think that doctors need to ask more questions": Sexual minority and majority adolescents' experiences talking about sexuality with healthcare providers. *Patient Education and Counseling, 99*(9), 1467–1472. https://doi.org/10.1016/j.pec.2016.06.004

Jarvis, C. (2020). *Physical examination & health assessment* (8th ed.). Saunders.

Kingsberg, S. A. (2006). Taking a sexual history. *Obstetrics and Gynecology Clinics, 33*(4), 535–547.

Lough, M. E., Shradar, E., Hsieh, C. & Hedlin, H. (2019). Contamination in adult midstream clean-catch urine cultures in the emergency department: A randomized controlled trial. *Journal of Emergency Nursing, 45*(5), 488–501. https://doi.org/10.1016/j.jen.2019.06.001

Matuszkiewicz-Rowińska, J., Małyszko, J., & Wieliczko, M. (2015). Urinary tract infections in pregnancy: Old and new unresolved diagnostic and therapeutic problems. *Archives of Medical Science, 11*(1), 67–77. https://doi.org/10.5114/aoms.2013.39202

Mishra, V., Singh, P., & Singh, L. M. (2018). Assessment of risk factors contributing to urinary tract infections in women. *International Journal of Medical Science and Clinical Invention, 5*(3), 3577–3579. https://doi.org/10.18535/ijmsci/v5i3.02

Nemours TeensHealth. (n.d.). *How can I see my doctor without my parents?* https://kidshealth.org/en/teens/doctor-alone.html

Potter, P. A., Perry, A. G., Stockert, P., & Hall, A. (2017). *Fundamentals of nursing* (9th ed.). Elsevier.

Santa Maria, D., Guilamo-Ramos, V., Jemmott, L. S., Derouin, A., & Villarruel, A. (2017). Nurses on the front lines: Improving adolescent sexual and reproductive health across health care settings. *American Journal of Nursing, 117*(1), 42–51. https://doi.org/10.1097/01.NAJ.0000511566.12446.45

Study.com. (n.d.). *The nine abdominal regions.* https://study.com/learn/lesson/regions-abdomen-overview-locations-nine.html

Thompson, J. M. (2018). Pain assessment. In J. M. Thompson (Ed.), *Essential health assessment* (pp. 91–103). F. A. Davis Company.

Thompson, J., & Scannell, M. (2018). Assessing the female breasts, axillae, and reproductive system. In J. M. Thompson (Ed.), *Essential health assessment* (pp. 311–342). F. A. Davis Company.

Urology Care Foundation. (2019). *Ask the experts: How do I know if I have a urinary tract infection (UTI)?* https://www.urologyhealth.org/patient-magazine/magazine-archives/2019/summer-2019/ask-the-experts-how-do-i-know-if-i-have-a-uti

Venes, D. (Ed.). (2013). *Taber's cyclopedic medical dictionary* (22nd ed.). F. A. Davis Company.

White, L. (2018). Assessment of the pregnant woman. In J. M. Thompson (Ed.), *Essential health assessment* (pp. 536–554). F. A. Davis Company.

CHAPTER 14

Dermatological Anomalies

Kristi Maynard, EdD, APRN, FNP-BC, CNE

 CASE STUDY

Patient Presenting to Clinic for Routine Physical Exam

- 61-year-old female
- No pressing health concerns

T 97.8°F oral	**HR** 74 bpm	**BP** 124/72	**RR** 12	**O2** 98%	**Pain** 0/10

Makayla is a 61-year-old Caucasian female who presents to the community health clinic for a routine physical examination. The nurse begins the process of obtaining a complete health history from Makayla before beginning the physical examination. The patient reveals she has no health concerns at this time and has been feeling "great." She has been working as a landscape designer and spends much of her time outdoors. She denies any significant past medical history. She denies any environmental or drug allergies. Her family history is significant for hypertension, with both her father and paternal grandfather receiving treatment to control their blood pressure.

QUESTION 14.1 (Multiple response)

When preparing to exam a patient's skin, the nurse understands: *(Select all that apply)*

- **A)** The skin is the smallest body organ.
- **B)** The skin is composed of three layers.
- **C)** The skin plays a major role in temperature regulation.
- **D)** The skin has sensory functions that protect the body.

Answer: B, C, D

RATIONALE

The skin is the largest organ of the body. It covers the equivalent of 22 square feet and has a total weight of approximately 8 pounds. Amazingly, the skin can completely replace itself every 28 days (Leen, 2017). The skin has many purposes: It helps provide structure and shape to our bodies, protects underlying structures, is a major contributor to the sensory interpretation of our surrounding environment, and aids in temperature regulation.

> *Melanin* is a dark brown to black pigment produced by melanocytes that develops when skin is exposed to sunlight to protect the skin from UV exposure (Das, 2022).

The skin is composed of three layers: the epidermis, the dermis, and the underlying subcutaneous or fatty layer (see Figure 14.1). The *epidermis* is the top layer of the skin; it is the layer you see. In some areas of the body, the epidermis can be extremely thin (e.g., over the eyelids), while in other areas, it may be very thick (e.g., on the soles of the feet). The epidermis has three primary functions (Benedetti, 2022):

- It makes new skin cells at the base, which gradually migrate to the top layer.
- It protects the body as part of the immune system.
- It gives the skin its color through the production of melanin.

The next layer of the skin, the *dermis,* has many functions. Sweat is produced in the dermal layer by eccrine and apocrine glands. Sweating, or perspiring, is a natural mechanism of temperature regulation. Sweat is excreted to the skin's surface when the body's temperature is increasing. These excretions evaporate and have a cooling effect, thereby reducing body temperature (Benedetti, 2022). Additional structures housed within the layers of the skin include nerve endings to conduct impulses that develop our sense of touch; hair follicles, which are responsible for hair growth that provides warmth and protection; arterial and venous vasculature to supply blood flow and oxygen to skin tissues; and oil glands that aid in maintaining skin hydration and integrity (American Skin Association, n.d.).

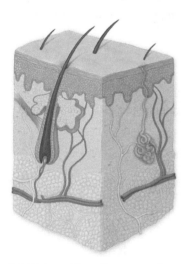

FIGURE 14.1 Normal cross-section of the skin in layers.

> **QUESTION 14.2 (Fill in the blank)**
>
> In considering Makayla's dermatological health, list three interview questions that should be included as part of her complete health history:
>
> 1. _____
>
> 2. _____
>
> 3. _____

ANSWER(S)/RATIONALE

The skin is a large and complex organ, so subjective data collection focused on the dermatological system must include interview questions that screen for pertinent family history, personal dermatological history, symptoms of current disease, potential harmful exposures, and relevant self-care behaviors. Some sample questions might include (Jarvis, 2016):

- Do you have a history of skin disease, allergies, hives, psoriasis, or eczema?
- Are you aware of any family history of skin disease, cancers, or related disorders?
- Have you noticed any changes in the skin, including changes in pigmentation or color, size, shape, or tenderness?
- Are you experiencing any excessive dryness or moisture?
- Are you experiencing any *pruritus* (skin itching)?
- Have you noticed excessive bruising?
- Have you noticed any rashes or lesions?
- Do you take any medications (prescription and over the counter)?
- Have you noticed any hair loss? Where?
- Have you noticed any change in nails' shape, color, or brittleness?
- Are you aware of any environmental or occupational exposures that may impact your dermatological health?
- What self-care behaviors do you regularly engage in? For example, applying sunscreen or the use of cleansers or moisturizers.

If appropriate, the nurse should further explore the patient's positive responses to include information on when the symptom began, where they noticed the change, if they have noticed anything that has made it better or worse, and if it has any associated symptoms.

QUESTION 14.3 (Multiple response)
Which of the following are risk factors for developing cancerous skin lesions?
(Select all that apply)

A) Ultraviolet light exposure   **D)** Frequent use of skin products

B) Age 20–30   **E)** Family history

C) Fair skin

Answer: A, C, E

 RATIONALE

There are three major types of skin cancer:

1. Basal cell carcinoma
2. Squamous cell carcinoma
3. Melanoma

Melanoma is the most serious form of skin cancer originating from melanocytes. According to the American Cancer Society (2023), risk factors for melanoma include:

Ultraviolet (UV) light exposure: UV rays originate from the sun. Without adequate protection, they have the capability to damage skin cell DNA, causing abnormal growth, as is the case in skin cancer.

Presence of atypical moles: Moles, known as *nevi*, are a normal, nonthreatening occurrence; however, if a person has more moles, they may be more likely to develop melanoma over the course of their life.

Fair skin: People with white skin are at the greatest risk of developing skin cancer. Fair-skinned people, especially those with red or blonde hair, green or blue eyes, freckling, or those who sunburn easily, are at the greatest risk; however, individuals of any skin tone can potentially develop skin cancer.

Family history: If a first-degree relative (a parent, sibling, or child) has had melanoma, the risk of developing the disease is higher. In fact, about 10% of patients diagnosed with melanoma have a family history of the disease.

Personal history of skin cancer: Someone who has already had a diagnosis of skin cancer is at an increased risk of developing a subsequent lesion.

Weakened immune system: Patients with weak immune systems are more likely to develop skin cancer. Conditions that may weaken the immune system include HIV or autoimmune diseases.

Advanced age: Skin cancer can occur at any age; however, the risk increases with age.

Gender: The risk is higher for women before the age of 50, but after age 50, the risk is higher in men.

Patient information continued... Makayla reveals that during an average workday, she will spend approximately six hours in direct sunlight. Although she does wear a wide-brimmed hat to prevent tan lines from her sunglasses, she does not employ any additional method of UV protection. She explains her natural skin tone is very pale and she likes to maintain a tan; she is worried that applying sunscreen will impact her ability to tan. With specific questioning, Makayla reports having a few moles on her upper back that "have been there forever" but denies any specific concerns regarding her skin.

QUESTION 14.4 (Multiple choice)

What statement by the patient demonstrates a need for further education regarding sun safety?

A) "My skin should be safe from sun damage. I wear SPF 25 sunscreen outdoors."

B) "There is no need to reapply sunscreen after I go for a swim."

C) "UV rays can damage the skin in as little as 15 minutes."

D) "I need to check the expiration date on my sunscreen before I use it."

Answer: B

RATIONALE

According to the Centers for Disease Control and Prevention (CDC), the sun's UV rays can damage the skin in as little as 15 minutes (CDC, 2023b). Some ways to prevent damage from UV rays include finding shade, wearing protective clothing and hats, and wearing sunscreen. Sunscreen is rated according to its sun protection factor (SPF). A minimum SPF of 15 is recommended; the higher the SPF, the more protection the product provides from the sun. Patients must be instructed to reapply the product per manufacturer recommendations or after swimming or sweating. Sunscreen expires, like most other health and beauty products, and may not be as potent if the product has expired. Although most sun care products have a shelf life of three years, exposure to heat can damage them (CDC, 2023b).

QUESTION 14.5 (Multiple choice)

With consideration to the patient's subjective history, the nurse is *most* concerned with an increased risk for:

A) Melanoma

B) Lentigo senilis

C) Tinea corporis

D) Candidiasis

E) Atopic dermatitis

Answer: A

RATIONALE

Melanoma risk would be the biggest concern for Makayla. She is a fair-skinned individual with a history of "moles" on the back and unprotected, daily exposure to the sun. Melanoma is the most aggressive form of skin cancer (Skin Cancer Foundation, 2022). A is the only option that can be potentially fatal while the others are common, treatable conditions.

Lentigo senilis is more commonly known as "liver spots" and is a normal variant of aging associated with changes in skin pigmentation that may develop over time as the result of UV exposure (see Figure 14.2). They are not considered to be dangerous lesions; they are usually a cosmetic nuisance (Mehregan, 1975).

Tinea corporis (ringworm) is a common fungal skin infection (see Figure 14.3). It is characterized as a dry, scaly rash that is usually round or ovoid in shape (Sahoo & Mahajan, 2016). The condition is treated with antifungal medication. Diagnosis of tinea may be confirmed with the use of a device called a woods lamp. A *woods lamp* uses blacklight and magnification to enhance the dermatological exam. Certain fungal infections like tinea may illuminate or glow when subjected to blacklight.

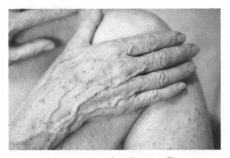

FIGURE 14.2 Lentigo senilis.

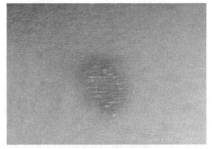

FIGURE 14.3 Tinea corporis.

Candidiasis is also a fungal infection caused by candida. Candida is most likely to grow in warm, moist areas such as under the breasts or in the folds of the abdomen. Candida is known for its erythematous, scaly appearance.

It can be treated with antifungal agents but can be resistant; therefore, good hygiene practices are critical to eradicate candida and prevent its return (Vergidis, 2023).

Atopic dermatitis, or eczema, is a condition caused by an abnormal immune response with exposure to sensitive allergens (see Figure 14.4). This leads to regional inflammation that produces an itchy, dry, scaly rash. While atopic dermatitis is genetically predetermined, minimizing the exposure to known irritants, such as extreme temperature or known environmental allergens, can reduce the incidence of rash.

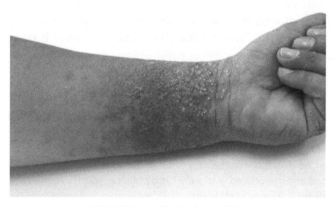

FIGURE 14.4 Atopic dermatitis.

Patient information continued… After collecting the complete health history, the nurse prepares Makayla for her physical exam and collects necessary equipment to complete the examination. He recognizes that, while most of the dermatological exam involves inspection, palpation techniques will also be utilized for a complete assessment.

QUESTION 14.6 (Multiple response)

When preparing for a dermatological exam, what supplies does the nurse gather? *(Select all that apply)*

A) Gloves

B) Floor lamp

C) Stethoscope

D) Ruler

E) Marking pen

Answer: A, B, D, E

RATIONALE

Gloves should be worn whenever you touch skin surfaces that are potentially disrupted to avoid contact with potentially transferrable diseases or body fluids. A second pair of gloves should be readily available in case you soil your initial pair. Adequate lighting is critical in performing a comprehensive assessment of the skin. Standard room lighting may be enhanced with the use of a magnified handheld light source or a bright floor lamp. Use caution when positioning light sources because bulbs may become hot, posing a risk to you and your patient. A ruler and marking pen are used to document identified lesions. Whenever a lesion is encountered, it should be measured for length and width in millimeters or centimeters and appropriately documented in the patient's chart. A magnifying glass may also be considered for skin examination to enlarge small lesions or infestations. A stethoscope is not imperative during the dermatological exam because there is no auscultation involved.

Patient information continued... The nurse begins the preliminary skin evaluation. He begins the exam by inspecting the hair. He uses a tongue blade to carefully separate the patient's hair into sections, allowing him to examine the scalp. Her hair color appears to be a natural blond with no evidence of thinning, alopecia, or scalp lesions. Next, the nurse moves on to examine the fingernails. The nails are well groomed and manicured with a dark red polish applied. When evaluating profile sign, there is no evidence of clubbing.

QUESTION 14.7 (Multiple choice)

Which of the following is a normal variant when examining a patient's hair?

A) Presence of nits　　　　**C)** Alopecia

B) White coloration　　　　**D)** Seborrheic dermatitis

Answer: B

RATIONALE

Hair naturally occurs in a variety of colors. As one ages, the production of pigment in the hair will begin to decline, resulting in gray or white hair color (Curley, 2020).

The term *nit* refers to eggs laid in the hair by head lice (*pediculus humanus capitis*). Head lice (see Figure 14.5) is a commonly occurring infestation that spreads rapidly from host to host. It is known to cause an itchy scalp and requires treatment for eradication (CDC, 2023a).

Alopecia is the technical term for hair loss. It can occur on any region of the body that is expected to have hair even though it is commonly associated with hair loss from the scalp. Alopecia can result from genetic influence or may be a consequence of certain diseases or medications; for example, chemotherapy is known to cause alopecia as it destroys the ability of hair cells to reproduce (Ludmann, 2023).

Seborrheic dermatitis, more commonly known as dandruff, is abnormal flaking of the scalp due to dryness or abnormalities with oil production (see Figure 14.6). It is a very common condition characterized by flakes of white or yellow skin from the scalp that shed or become stuck in the hair (Mayo Clinic, 2022).

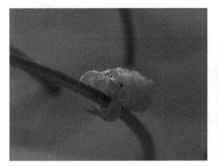
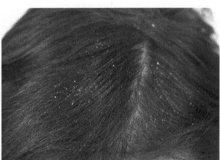

FIGURE 14.5 Head louse.   FIGURE 14.6 Dandruff.

QUESTION 14.8 (Multiple choice)

When describing appropriate technique for assessing the fingernails, the nurse is correct in stating:

A) Nail polish must be removed to facilitate a complete exam.

B) Profile sign is performed when the nail of the fifth digit is observed from a lateral view.

C) Capillary refill indicates a patient's hydration status.

D) The nails provide minimal information on a patient's health status.

Answer: A

RATIONALE

The fingernails provide a lot of information about a patient's health status. Hypoxemia, nutritional deficiencies, and circulatory anomalies can be appreciated through examination of the nails (Mayo Clinic, 2023). To facilitate a comprehensive examination of the nails, nail polish should be completely removed. Doing so will reveal the nail beds and growth plates, making variants such as color changes (e.g., cyanosis), ridges, or lesions more apparent.

Profile sign is a test used to determine the presence of nail clubbing. Clubbing occurs when the patient is in a chronic hypoxic state, as might be the case in chronic obstructive pulmonary disease. Profile sign is performed when a lateral view of the index finger is observed to evaluate the angle of the nail plate. Normally, the angle of the nail plate should be 160° or less. If the angle is greater than 160°, clubbing is present. Schamroth's sign (see Figure 14.7) is another method to evaluate for clubbing (Agarwal et al., 2019).

The Schamroth Window Test

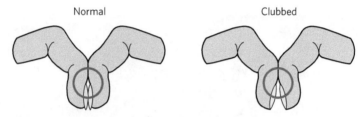

Normal   Clubbed

FIGURE 14.7 Schamroth's sign.

Capillary refill is an assessment of perfusion. It is performed by placing pressure on the nail bed to cause a blanched appearance. When pressure is released, pink coloration should return to the nail bed within three seconds. If it takes longer than three seconds for color to return, it may be assumed there is compromised or sluggish blood flow to the extremity.

Patient information continued... The nurse has completed his examination of the hair and nails and prepares to examine the skin. The patient is comfortably seated on the exam table dressed in a gown. The room has ample lighting, and a floor lamp is available if needed. Initial inspection of the exposed skin on the arms reveals even coloration with no evidence of erythema, cyanosis, or pallor. Hyperpigmented patches are present on the posterior aspect of each hand. Otherwise, the exposed skin surfaces are intact with no remarkable findings.

QUESTION 14.9 (Multiple choice)

While examining the patient's skin, the nurse appreciates a slight bluish tint that is more pronounced around the mouth and nail beds. The nurse would document this variant as:

A) Pallor   **B)** Jaundice   **C)** Cyanosis   **D)** Erythema

Answer: C

RATIONALE

Cyanosis is a blue discoloration of the skin that signifies poor perfusion or hypoxemia. It is a sign that the patient is not receiving adequate oxygenation. Cyanosis is more pronounced around the mouth or mucous membranes and the nail beds, and it produces a bluish discoloration in patients with light skin tones. In patients with darker skin tones, cyanosis might appear as a grayish-white discoloration around the mouth or a dark, maroon coloration of the nail beds. It is best to assess for cyanosis in low pigment areas such as the oral mucosa, sclera, or nail bed.

Jaundice describes a yellowish discoloration of the skin and sclera that develops as the result of elevated levels of bilirubin. We typically associate the presence of jaundice with liver disease.

Pallor describes pale or blanched skin and may be caused by conditions such as anemia or shock. For all skin tones, pallor is best appreciated by assessing the oral mucosa or conjunctiva.

Erythema is typically used to describe redness; however, patients with dark skin tones might develop a deep purple discoloration in areas of injury or inflammation. Since the presentation of erythema can vary, the nurse should palpate for temperature when inflammation or injury is suspected to correlate changes in coloration to changes in temperature (Sommers, 2011). Should you assess a structure that displays erythema, it is said to be erythematous.

QUESTION 14.10 (Fill in the blank)

List three qualities of the skin the nurse might appreciate with initial inspection and palpation:

1. _____

2. _____

3. _____

ANSWER(S)/RATIONALE

Although the examination of the skin may seem simple, it is actually quite complex. Skin qualities you will assess utilizing techniques of inspection and palpation are included in Table 14.1.

TABLE 14.1 Skin Assessment Descriptors

Quality	Common Descriptors
Color	Consistent, cyanotic, erythematous, jaundice, flushed
Moisture	Dry, diaphoretic, clammy
Texture	Rough, smooth, hydrated, coarse
Thickness	Appropriate for age, thin
Edema/swelling	Pitting, nonpitting, graded 0–4
Mobility	Mobile, scarred, contracted
Vascularity	Prominent vasculature, ecchymosis, vascular lesions

---

QUESTION 14.11 (Multiple choice)

The nurse informs his patient that he will be palpating for skin turgor. Skin turgor evaluates a patient's:

A) Hydration status

B) Collagen deposits

C) Temperature

D) Skin mobility

Answer: A

RATIONALE

Skin turgor is a measure of hydration status. Turgor is evaluated by pinching the skin directly below the clavicle or on the posterior aspect of the hand. As the skin is pinched, it "tents"; this tenting should rebound to its normal position when released. If the skin remains in a tented position, it is an indicator of dehydration. The clavicle is the preferred site to evaluate turgor because the skin of the back of the hand may be more likely to remain tented as a normal variant of age as elasticity is lost over time (Kaneshiro, 2023).

QUESTION 14.12 (Multiple choice)

The nurse examining Makayla documents hyperpigmented patches present on the posterior aspect of each hand. Which of the following is an expected variant when examining the skin of an older adult?

A) Increased elasticity

B) Oily skin

C) Increased capillary fragility

D) Increased melanocyte function

Answer: C

RATIONALE

The older adult is more likely to experience increased capillary fragility, which leads to leaking into the skin tissues. These "leaks" are hyperpigmented lesions commonly recognized as *senile purpura* or liver spots (Kuter, 2023). The other options are the opposite of the expected dermatological changes with aging. Look at the image in Figure 14.8 and compare the hand of the younger adult to the older adult; what are some obvious differences you can spot?

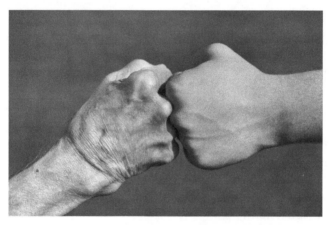

FIGURE 14.8 Comparison of skin qualities across the life span.

Some common changes you may appreciate with the elder population may include (Tobin et al., 2017):

- Loss of skin elasticity (skin begins to fold and sag)
- Decrease in number and function of sweat and sebaceous glands (causing skin to become drier)
- Increased risk of skin breakdown due to slower cell replacement and delayed wound healing
- Changes in hair matrix secondary to decreased functioning melanocytes in the hair (leading to gray and fine hair)

Patient information continued... After inspecting and palpating the exposed surfaces of the skin, the nurse repositions the drape to expose the skin of the back. He notices four moles on the upper back. One of the moles stands out from the others. It is large, the coloring is a reddish-brown, and the borders appear rough and irregular.

QUESTION 14.13 **(Multiple choice)**

The appropriate terminology to describe a hyperpigmented, flat skin lesion commonly known as a "mole" is:

A) Macule

B) Papule

C) Vesicle

D) Plaque

Answer: A

RATIONALE

When describing a skin lesion, it is critical that proper terminology is used for the sake of professionalism and continuity in documentation. The term to describe a mole is a *nevus,* which is further classified as a *macule* as long as there is no appreciated elevation. If the lesion is elevated, it may be considered a *papule.* Lesions are separated into two categories: primary and secondary skin lesions. Primary skin lesions arise from a specific causative factor, while secondary lesions result from the evolution of a primary lesion. For example, if a patient has an itchy mosquito bite, the bite is a *wheal,* a type of primary lesion, and the scratch marks from frequent itching would be a secondary lesion. Table 14.2 highlights some of the more common terms used to describe skin lesions.

TABLE 14.2 Primary Skin Lesions

Lesion	Description	Example
Macule	Flat, circumscribed, less than 1 cm	Freckle, small nevus
Papule	Solid, elevated, circumscribed, less than 1 cm	Wart
Vesicle	Fluid-filled blister up to 1 cm	Chicken pox, poison ivy
Bulla	Fluid-filled blister larger than 1 cm	Blister
Patch	Flat, circumscribed, greater than 1 cm	Café au lait spot
Cyst	Encapsulated, fluid-filled cavity	Cystic acne
Wheal	Superficial, raised, transient, erythematous	Mosquito bite, urticaria

(Jarvis, 2016)

QUESTION 14.14 (Fill in the blank)
When evaluating a skin lesion's likelihood of being cancerous, the mnemonic ABCDE is used. What does ABCDE stand for?

A. _____

B. _____

C. _____

D. _____

E. _____

F. _____

Answer: A. Asymmetry; B. Border; C. Color; D. Diameter; E. Elevation

RATIONALE
The ABCDE mnemonic stands for:

A: Asymmetry—If you were to fold the lesion in half, would the edges match? If not, the lesion is said to be asymmetrical. Asymmetry is concerning for malignancy.

B: Border—The border should appear smooth and consistent. Rough, irregular borders would be worrisome.

C: Color—Is the color of the lesion consistent throughout? If the coloration is inconsistent or contains different pigments, it would be considered suspicious.

D: Diameter—Is the lesion greater than 6 mm?

E: Elevation, enlargement, or evolution—Is the lesion raised? Or has the lesion enlarged or evolved? Change or growth may be a sign of malignancy (Duate et al., 2021).

Review Figure 14.9 and apply what you know about ABCDE screening. This is an example of melanoma; you can recognize the asymmetric appearance, irregular border, and inconsistent coloration. Based on these findings, this patient would require a referral for further evaluation of the lesion.

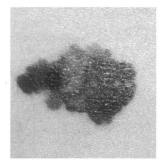

FIGURE 14.9 Skin cancer.

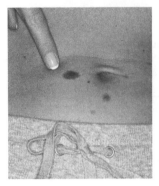

FIGURE 14.10 Ugly duckling.

A method you may use when evaluating the skin is the "ugly duckling rule." This may be particularly helpful if a patient has multiple skin lesions. According to the ugly duckling rule, we pay special attention to lesions that are distinctly different from the others—they stand out (Jensen & Elewski, 2015).

When looking at Figure 14.10, the large lesion to the left of the umbilicus has different qualities than the other lesions on the abdomen. It is obviously larger, has inconsistent coloration, is asymmetric, and has irregular borders.

Patient information continued… The nurse completed the skin assessment. He discusses his findings with Makayla and informs her that he will be placing a referral for her to consult with a dermatologist due to the irregular nevus noted on her upper back.

QUESTION 14.15 (Short answer)

Based on Makayla's presentation, why do you think a referral is being made?

_____

_____

_____

_____

ANSWER/RATIONALE

Makayla is being referred because of the presence of a suspicious skin lesion. Lesions suspected to be malignant require prompt evaluation that may include biopsy. In addition to evaluating her skin lesion, a comprehensive skin evaluation by a dermatologist would be advisable considering her fair skin and history of excessive sun exposure. Routine dermatological assessments are critical for the early identification and treatment of malignant lesions.

QUESTION 14.16 (Short answer)

What are three patient teaching topics that should be included during Makayla's visit?

1. _____

2. _____

3. _____

 ANSWER(S)/RATIONALE

Some pertinent teaching points may include:

1. Use of sunscreen and how to protect the skin from UV exposure
2. Recommendations for annual skin checks by a licensed dermatological provider
3. Frequent self-evaluation of skin integrity for early identification of suspicious lesions
4. How to use the ABCDE screening for self-skin checks
5. The different types of skin cancer
6. Common risk factors

CHAPTER 14 WORKSHEET

Based on my initial assessment, I thought:

_____

_____

_____

Based on my revised/informed assessment, I now know:

_____

_____

_____

A nursing priority for this patient would be _____

because _____

After completing this chapter, something I have learned is:

_____

_____

_____

After completing this chapter, something I need more clarity on is:

_____

_____

_____

After completing this chapter, something else I want to learn is:

_____

_____

_____

REFERENCES

Agarwal, R., Baid, R., & Sinha, D. P. (2019). Clubbing: The oldest clinical sign in medicine. *CHRISMED Journal of Health and Research*, 6(1), 72.

American Cancer Society. (2023). *Risk factors for melanoma skin cancer.* https://www.cancer.org/cancer/melanoma-skin-cancer/causes-risks-prevention/risk-factors.html

American Skin Association. (n.d.). *Healthy skin.* http://www.americanskin.org/resource/

Benedetti, J. (2022). Structure and function of the skin. *Merck Manual.* https://www.merckmanuals.com/home/skin-disorders/biology-of-the-skin/structure-and-function-of-the-skin

Centers for Disease Control and Prevention. (2023a). *Head lice.* https://www.cdc.gov/parasites/lice/head/index.html

Centers for Disease Control and Prevention. (2023b). *Sun safety.* https://www.cdc.gov/cancer/skin/basic_info/sun-safety.htm

Curley, C. (2020). *Scientists think they know how stress causes gray hair.* https://www.healthline.com/health-news/scientists-how-stress-causes-gray-hair

Das, S. (2022). Overview of skin pigment. *Merck Manual.* https://www.merckmanuals.com/home/skin-disorders/pigment-disorders/overview-of-skin-pigment

Duarte, A. F., Sousa-Pinto, B., Azevedo, L. F., Barros, A. M., Puig, S., Malvehy, J., Haneke, E., & Correia, O. (2021). Clinical ABCDE rule for early melanoma detection. *European Journal of Dermatology*, 31(6), 771-778.

Jarvis, C. (2016). *Physical examination & health assessment* (7th ed.). Saunders.

Jensen, J. D., & Elewski, B. E. (2015). The ABCDEF rule: Combining the "ABCDE rule" and the "ugly duckling sign" in an effort to improve patient self-screening examinations. *The Journal of Clinical and Aesthetic Dermatology*, 8(2), 15.

Kaneshiro, N. K. (2023). *Skin turgor.* https://medlineplus.gov/ency/imagepages/17223.htm

Kuter, D. J. (2023). Senile purpura. *Merck Manual Professional Version.* https://www.merckmanuals.com/professional/hematology-and-oncology/bleeding-due-to-abnormal-blood-vessels/senile-purpura

Leen, S. (2017, Jan. 17). Skin. *National Geographic.* https://www.nationalgeographic.com/science/health-and-human-body/human-body/skin

Ludmann, P. (2023). *Alopecia areata.* American Academy of Dermatology Associates. https://www.aad.org/public/diseases/hair-loss/types/alopecia

Mayo Clinic. (2022). *Seborrheic dermatitis.* https://www.mayoclinic.org/diseases-conditions/seborrheic-dermatitis/symptoms-causes/syc-20352710

Mayo Clinic. (2023). *7 fingernail problems not to ignore.* https://www.mayoclinic.org/healthy-lifestyle/adult-health/multimedia/nails/sls-20076131?s=2

Mehregan, A. H. (1975). Lentigo senilis and its evolutions. *Journal of Investigative Dermatology*, 65(5), 429–433.

Sahoo, A. K., & Mahajan, R. (2016). Management of tinea corporis, tinea cruris, and tinea pedis: A comprehensive review. *Indian Dermatology Online Journal*, 7(2), 77–86.

Skin Cancer Foundation. (2022). *Melanoma overview.* https://www.skincancer.org/skin-cancer-information/melanoma/

Sommers, M. S. (2011, Jan. 11). Color awareness: A must for patient assessment. *American Nurse.* https://www.myamericannurse.com/color-awareness-a-must-for-patient-assessment/

Tobin, D. J., Veysey, E. C., & Finlay, A. Y. (2017). Aging and the skin. In H. M. Fillit, K. Rockword, & J. Young (Eds.), *Brocklehurst's textbook of geriatric medicine and gerontology* (8th ed.). Elsevier.

Vergidis, P. (2023). Candidiasis. *Merck Manual Professional Version.* https://www.merckmanuals.com/professional/infectious-diseases/fungi/candidiasis

Head and Neck Anomalies

Kristi Maynard, EdD, APRN, FNP-BC, CNE

CASE STUDY

Patient Presenting to Outpatient Clinic With Sinus Infection

- 32-year-old female
- 10-day history of headache, fever, nasal discharge

| **T** 100.2°F oral | **HR** 72 bpm | **BP** 128/74 | **RR** 14 | **O2** 98% | **Pain** 6/10 |

Jordan is a 32-year-old female who presents to the outpatient clinic today concerned that she has developed a sinus infection. She has had symptoms of headache, fever, and purulent nasal discharge for about 10 days. Her symptoms began after her flight home from vacation and have been getting progressively worse. She denies any medication or environmental allergies. Her current medications include sertraline for the treatment of depression, which she started about six months ago, and a daily multivitamin.

QUESTION 15.1 (Multiple choice)

The patient presents with a possible sinus infection. What are three subjective questions the nurse should ask to collect focused data for this visit?

1. _____

2. _____

3. _____

ANSWER(S)/RATIONALE

When collecting a focused history, you are only looking to obtain information relevant to the presenting complaint. It may be useful to use the PQRSTU mnemonic to guide your subjective questioning. While this mnemonic is traditionally used for pain, it can be modified to guide questioning for other presenting symptoms or conditions. Using this method to guide your questioning, pertinent subjective questions for the presenting complaint might include:

P: Provocation/Palliation—Have you noticed anything that makes your symptoms better or worse?

Q: Quality—What symptoms are you having? How would you describe them?

R: Region or Radiation—Where do you feel the discomfort? Are there any associated symptoms?

S: Severity Scale—On a scale of 0 to 10, how much has the condition interrupted your daily life? How so? (You may also choose to use the standard 0 to 10 scale to assess pain if it is reported with the chief complaint.)

T: Timing—When did your symptoms begin? If they come and go, how long do they last?

U: Understanding—What do you think it may be?

(Crozer Health, n.d.)

QUESTION 15.2 (Multiple response)

Which of the following are facial sinuses? *(Select all that apply)*

A) Ethmoid   **D)** Sphenoid

B) Mandibular   **E)** Frontal

C) Maxillary

Answer: A, C, D, E

RATIONALE

There are four paired sinuses in the face: The frontal sinuses are found in the forehead, the ethmoid and sphenoid are behind the nose, and the maxillary are located at the medial aspect of the cheekbones (Cleveland Clinic, n.d.). *Sinuses* are air-spaced cavities in the skull; they help in reducing the overall weight of the skull by reducing the amount of solid bone. They are also known to improve the quality of our voices through resonance, but most importantly, they assist in normal mucous production for the nose (Cedars Sinai, n.d.). When sinus cavities become infected, symptoms might include discolored nasal discharge, nasal congestion, facial tenderness, headaches, pain in the teeth, foul breath, and fever. While many sinus infections are caused by viruses, others may be caused by bacteria or fungi. Early identification of bacterial and fungal infections is important to prevent the illness from spreading to other regional structures including the facial bones and brain (American College of Allergy, Asthma, & Immunology, n.d.).

Patient information continued... In addition to the headaches, Jordan is also concerned with a feeling of "fullness" in the right ear. This began seven days after her symptoms started. A muffled sensation is associated with the fullness. She denies any pain or drainage in the ear.

QUESTION 15.3 (Multiple choice)

When performing an exam of the external ear structure, the nurse inspects the:

A) Helix, tragus, and mastoid

B) Malleus, incus, and stapes

C) Lacrimal duct, sclera, and palpebral fissure

D) Ear canal, cerumen, and hair follicles

Answer: A

RATIONALE

The helix, tragus, and mastoid are major structures of the external ear. The *external ear* is the portion of the ear that can be easily viewed on the outside of the body with no special equipment (see Figure 15.1). The mastoid is located behind the ear in the region of the mastoid process of the skull. Inflammation or pain at this location may indicate a condition known as mastoiditis, which usually occurs as the result of untreated *otitis media* (middle ear infection). The external ear should be inspected and palpated prior to initiating any internal exam to evaluate for signs of infection or pain (Jan, 2024).

The malleus, incus, and stapes are the tiny bones or *ossicles* that are located in the middle ear behind the protective *tympanic membrane* (eardrum). They help to transmit sound (Stanford Children's Health, n.d.).

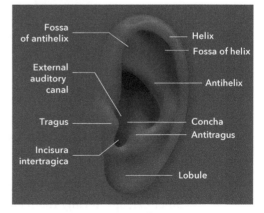

FIGURE 15.1 External ear structure.

QUESTION 15.4 (Multiple choice)

The tympanic membrane is the membrane that separates the external ear canal from the middle ear. A healthy tympanic membrane appears:

A) Erythematous, opaque

B) Gray, pearly

C) Clear, transparent

D) White, opaque

Answer: B

RATIONALE

A healthy tympanic membrane is translucent with a pearly, gray coloration. If the membrane has a red or erythematous appearance, the examiner would suspect possible irritation or infection. White coloration indicates thickening of the membrane, which may occur as the result of scarring. In the older adult, a white discoloration may be a normal variation, as sclerosis (hardening) of the membrane may occur (Jarvis, 2016).

Aside from coloration, a healthy tympanic membrane should have certain identifiable landmarks. When using an *otoscope* (the lighted device used to evaluate the ear; see Figure 15.2) to evaluate the tympanic membrane, the light of the scope should produce a reflection in the membrane. This reflection is known as the *cone of light*. The cone of light should be in the 5 o'clock position in the right ear and 7 o'clock position in the left. If the cone of light is absent or displaced, it indicates an abnormal shape or curvature of the tympanic membrane (Jarvis, 2016).

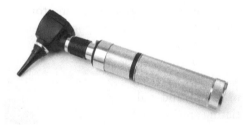

FIGURE 15.2 Otoscope.

The membrane is normally positioned in a slightly convex, neutral position (see Figure 15.3). If that position is exaggerated, it is said to be *bulging*. If the membrane pulls inward toward the middle ear, it is said to be *convex* or *retracted*. Either deformity may result from infections or scarring. In addition to the cone of light, the examiner can identify the outline of the bones of the inner ear, specifically the incus and malleus, through the membrane (Jarvis, 2016).

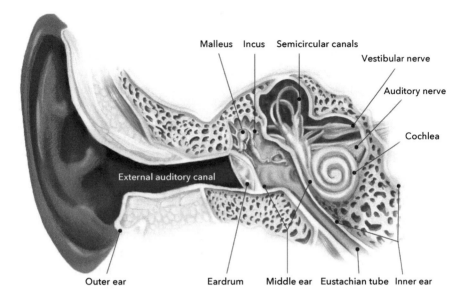

Malleus Incus Semicircular canals

Vestibular nerve

Auditory nerve

Cochlea

External auditory canal

Outer ear   Eardrum   Middle ear Eustachian tube Inner ear

FIGURE 15.3 Structures of the ear.

Patient information continued... The nurse proceeds to perform a preliminary ear, nose, and throat examination. The sinuses are notable for pressure and pain with palpation of the frontal and right maxillary sinus. The nasal mucosa is edematous and erythematous with evidence of thick, green, purulent discharge. There is no evidence of erosions in the nasal cavity. The right tympanic membrane appears gray and dull with evidence of serous effusion. Examination of the mouth and throat reveals an unremarkable oral cavity with evidence of good hydration and dentation. The posterior pharynx is slightly erythematous, tonsils are surgically absent, and patient confirms removal at the age of 6.

QUESTION 15.5 (Multiple choice)

When positioning the adult patient's ear for internal inspection, the nurse is correct when:

A) Pulling the helix down and out

B) Applying pressure to the tragus

C) No special positioning is necessary.

D) Pulling the helix up and back

Answer: D

RATIONALE

When positioning an adult patient for otoscopic examination, the examiner should place the head in a neutral position and pull the helix up and back. This action straightens the ear canal, thereby facilitating the internal exam. When planning to perform an internal otoscopic examination, a visual inspection of the ear canal should be performed first to ensure there is no foreign body or severe external canal infection that may be exacerbated with placement of the speculum. The painful ear should be evaluated last (Jarvis, 2016).

For small children, the ear would be appropriately positioned by pulling the helix down and back. The ear canals of small children are generally shorter and more curved than their adult counterparts (Jarvis, 2016). When working with children, it may be helpful to have the child seated in their caregiver's lap with the caregiver hugging the child's arms. This helps to reduce movement and prevents the child from reaching for the otoscope during the exam. The examiner must be aware of the possibility of sudden movement and position the otoscope accordingly to compensate for slight changes in head position. Insertion of the otoscope speculum (plastic cover) too far can cause damage to the tympanic membrane or ear canal.

QUESTION 15.6 (Multiple choice)

The patient presents complaining of decreased ability to hear. Which of the following would be most appropriate for the nurse to perform in the outpatient setting to evaluate for hearing loss?

A) Whisper test

B) Rinne and Weber test

C) Snellen chart

D) Audiometric evaluation

Answer: A

RATIONALE

The *whisper test* is the simplest, most efficient means of evaluating for hearing loss in the outpatient environment. To perform the whisper test, the examiner stands 2 feet behind the patient so that they are unable to read the examiner's lips. The examiner will instruct the patient to occlude the opposite of the ear they are testing, and then the examiner will whisper a series of three random, one-syllable words (usually letters or numbers) and ask the patient to repeat them back. If the patient is unsuccessful, a new series of words will be whispered during a repeat test. A second failure indicates likely hearing loss. The process is repeated on the opposite ear (Dick, 2018).

The Rinne and Weber exams utilize a tuning fork to assess for signs of conductive versus sensorineural hearing loss. Though these tests may still be seen in practice, they have come under fire for poor sensitivity (McGurgan & Nicholl, 2017). The Snellen chart is used to assess vision. Finally, audiometric testing is an acceptable (and usually preferred) means to evaluate for hearing loss; however, specialty equipment and training are required to perform this exam. Typically, if a patient has a strong suspicion of hearing loss or they fail a whisper test, they will be referred for more in-depth evaluation utilizing audiometric testing.

QUESTION 15.7 (Multiple choice)

Jordan's tonsils are noted to be surgically absent. If the tonsils were present and noted to be touching, the tonsils would be graded as:

A) Grade 1+   **B)** Grade 2+   **C)** Grade 3+   **D)** Grade 4+

Answer: D

RATIONALE

The *Brodsky grading scale* is one of the most common tools used to describe tonsil size. If the tonsils are absent due to surgical removal, it is appropriate to document "surgically absent." Otherwise, documentation follows the guidelines outlined in Table 15.1.

TABLE 15.1 Brodsky Grading Scale for Tonsil Size

Grade	Description
0	Tonsils within the tonsillar fossa
1+	Tonsils just outside of the tonsillar fossa occupying < 25% of the oropharyngeal width
2+	Tonsils occupy 26%–50% oropharyngeal width
3+	Tonsils occupy 51%–75% oropharyngeal width
4+	Tonsils occupy > 75% oropharyngeal width

(Ng et al., 2010)

QUESTION 15.8 (Multiple choice)

When describing the proper approach for assessing the facial sinuses, the nurse correctly states:

A) "I will use my thumbs to apply gentle pressure over the frontal and maxillary sinuses."

B) "I will use my penlight to transilluminate the ethmoid sinus."

C) "I will inspect for swelling over the cheekbones."

D) "I will auscultate the sinus cavity for evidence of fluid movement."

Answer: A

RATIONALE

Evaluation of the frontal and maxillary sinuses is performed using palpation (see Figure 15.4). The examiner uses the pads of the thumbs to apply gentle, steady pressure to the sinus. It is a positive finding if the patient reports increased pain or pressure with palpation.

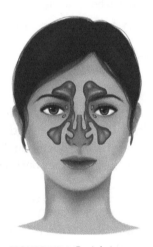

FIGURE 15.4 Facial sinuses.

Transillumination is a method traditionally used to assess for fluid or mucous consolidation within the frontal or maxillary sinuses; due to the placement of the ethmoid sinuses, transillumination cannot be performed. Transillumination is performed by placing the penlight against the skin over the sinus cavity to evaluate for the presence of opacity. If the light shines back red, there is no evidence of consolidation. If the light is dull, there is likely consolidation. Transillumination may be used to supplement the sinus exam but is no longer considered specific or sensitive enough to support diagnosis (Low et al., 1997).

Patient information continued... The nurse begins assessment of the regional lymph nodes. When palpating the lymph chains of the neck, she notices a prominent mass over the trachea. The nurse further assesses this mass by performing palpation of the thyroid gland.

QUESTION 15.9 (Multiple choice)

The nurse is assessing the regional lymph nodes of the head and neck. When palpating, what would be considered a "normal" finding?

A) Firm, immobile, painless lymph nodes

B) Soft, mobile, painless lymph nodes

C) Firm, mobile, painful lymph nodes

D) Soft, immobile, painful lymph nodes

Answer: B

RATIONALE

Lymph nodes are small structures of the immune system that promote drainage of lymphatic materials (see Table 15.2 and Figure 15.5). A normal lymph node can be up to 1 cm in diameter and is described as soft and mobile, meaning it is easily manipulated by the fingertips (Ferrer, 1998). In the absence of regional infection, nodes are usually painless; however, they may become tender as a normal variant if they are actively involved in fighting infection. Nodes that are firm, immobile, and painless should be considered abnormal and have a high suspicion for malignancy.

There are numerous lymph node chains and clusters distributed in the head and neck. When documenting your findings as they relate to the lymphatic system, you should specify the region where the abnormality was felt. *Lymphadenopathy* is the term used to describe enlarged or abnormal lymph nodes.

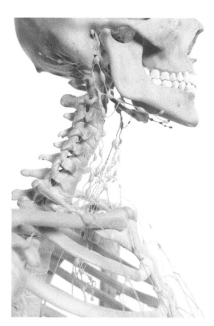

FIGURE 15.5 Regional lymph nodes.

TABLE 15.2 Lymph Nodes of the Head and Neck

Node	Location
Preauricular	In front of the ear
Posterior auricular	Superficial to the mastoid process
Occipital	Base of the skull
Submental	Midline behind the mandible
Submandibular	Halfway between the angle and the tip of the mandible
Jugulodigastric	Under the angle of the mandible
Superficial cervical	Overlying the sternomastoid muscle
Deep cervical	Under the sternomastoid muscle
Posterior cervical	Posterior triangle along the edge of the trapezius muscle
Supraclavicular	Above the clavicle

(Jarvis, 2016)

QUESTION 15.10 (Fill in the blank)

The nurse positions her hands for a thyroid examination with a posterior approach. Once she has identified landmarks and her hands are in place, she advises the patient to _____ .

A) Cough

B) Swallow

C) Turn her head from side to side

D) Say "Ah"

Answer: B

RATIONALE

The *thyroid gland* (see Figure 15.6) is critical for the production of hormones responsible for metabolism, growth, and development (National Center for Biotechnology Information, 2018). A thyroid exam can be performed using either an anterior or posterior approach. To employ the anterior approach, the patient should be examined in the seated or standing position. Locate the thyroid isthmus by palpating between the cricoid cartilage and the suprasternal notch. Then, using one hand, slightly retract the sternocleidomastoid muscle while palpating the thyroid with the other. Have the patient take a sip of water and swallow as you palpate. The thyroid will move upward under the fingertips (University of Washington Department of Medicine, n.d.).

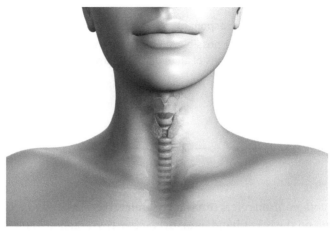

FIGURE 15.6 The thyroid gland.

The posterior approach is similar except you will position yourself behind the patient, and after locating the gland, move your hands laterally to try to feel under the sternocleidomastoid muscles to evaluate thyroid size (University of Washington Department of Medicine, n.d.). The examiner positioning can be seen in Figure 15.7.

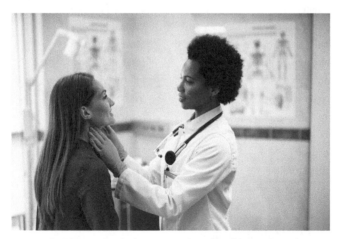

FIGURE 15.7 Posterior approach to thyroid assessment.

Patient information continued... Thyroid enlargement is confirmed with palpation. Review of the patient's medical record reveals a 30-pound weight gain over the past six months. With further questioning, Jordan admits she has been feeling more fatigued lately but assumed it was because of a change in her job schedule. Her hair appears coarse, and her skin is dry and flaking.

QUESTION 15.11 (Multiple response)

When evaluating a patient for possible hypothyroidism, the nurse recognizes which of the following to be signs of an underactive thyroid? *(Select all that apply)*

A) Dry hair

B) Weight gain

C) Heat intolerance

D) Bulging eyes

E) Fatigue

Answer: A, B, E

RATIONALE

Hypothyroidism refers to a state of underactive thyroid function; *hyperthyroidism,* on the other hand, is an overactive thyroid. See Table 15.3.

TABLE 15.3 Thyroid Dysfunction

Hypothyroidism	Hyperthyroidism
Dry hair	Hair loss
Puffy face	Bulging eyes
Slow heartbeat	Sweating
Weight gain	Elevated heartbeat
Constipation	Weight loss
Brittle nails	Sleep disturbances
Joint pain/muscle aches	Heat intolerance
Cold intolerance	Infertility
Depressed mood	Irritability
Dry skin	Muscle fatigue
Fatigue	Anxiety
Memory loss	
Heavy menstruation	

(Mayo Clinic, 2022)

QUESTION 15.12 Multiple choice)

With discovery of thyroid enlargement, what is another assessment technique the nurse may choose to perform to further evaluate the gland?

A) Percussion for thyroid borders

B) Palpation for regional lymph node inflammation

C) Auscultation for bruit

D) Inspection of the pharynx

Answer: C

RATIONALE

With thyroid enlargement, particularly with *Grave's disease,* which is a form of hyperthyroidism, it is possible for a bruit to develop due to the pro-liferation of additional blood vasculature (Williams et al., 2014). A *bruit* is a "whooshing" sound caused by increased, turbulent blood flow. When auscultating for a bruit, use the bell of the stethoscope. The other options are not part of the thyroid exam (Barnes, 1980).

Patient information continued... The physician confirms the nurse's exam findings. Based on her physical assessment, Jordan is determined to have bacterial sinusitis and is prescribed an appropriate antibiotic. In addition, the physician orders lab work for thyroid function.

Jordan follows up in the office one week later. Upon presentation, her sinusitis has resolved. Her lab work is significant for hypothyroidism. She is prescribed medication to normalize her thyroid values.

QUESTION 15.13 (Fill in the blank)

Considering Jordan's initial presentation, what are three signs (subjective or objective) that her thyroid function has improved?

1. _____

2. _____

3. _____

ANSWER(S)/RATIONALE

Jordan initially presented with weight gain, fatigue, coarse hair, and dry skin. Her medication history reveals she has been taking antidepressant medications. All these signs and symptoms are potentially caused by Jordan's underactive thyroid and would likely resolve with appropriate medical therapy.

CHAPTER 15 WORKSHEET

Based on my initial assessment, I thought:

_____

_____

_____

Based on my revised/informed assessment, I now know:

_____

_____

_____

A nursing priority for this patient would be _____

because _____

After completing this chapter, something I have learned is:

_____

_____

_____

After completing this chapter, something I need more clarity on is:

_____

_____

_____

After completing this chapter, something else I want to learn is:

_____

_____

_____

REFERENCES

American College of Allergy, Asthma, & Immunology. (n.d.). *Sinus infection.* https://acaai.org/allergies/types/sinus-infection

Barnes, R. W. (1980). Noninvasive evaluation of the carotid bruit. *Annual Review of Medicine, 31,* 201–218.

Cedars Sinai. (n.d.). *Sinus.* https://www.cedars-sinai.org/programs/ear-nose-throat/specialties/sinus.html

Cleveland Clinic. (n.d.). *Sinus infection.* https://my.clevelandclinic.org/health/diseases/17701-sinusitis

Dick, F. (2018). The whisper test and speech recognition tests. *Occupational Medicine, 68*(7), 488–489.

Ferrer, R. L. (1998). Lymphadenopathy: Differential diagnosis and evaluation. *American Family Physician, 58*(6), 1313–1320.

Jan, T. A. (2024). Mastoiditis. *Merck Manual Professional Version.* https://www.merckmanuals.com/professional/ear,-nose,-and-throat-disorders/middle-ear-and-tympanic-membrane-disorders/mastoiditis?query=mastoiditis

Jarvis, C. (2016). *Physical examination and health assessment.* (7th ed.). Saunders.

Low, D. E., Desrosiers, M., McSherry, J., Garber, G., Williams Jr, J. W., Rémy, H., Fenton, R. S., Forte, V., Balter, M., Rotstein, C., Craft, C., Dubois, J., Harding, G., Schloss, M., Miller, M., McIvor, R. A., & Davidson, R. J. (1997). A practical guide for the diagnosis and treatment of acute sinusitis. *Canadian Medical Association Journal, 156*(6), S1–14.

Mayo Clinic. (2022). *Hyperthyroidism (overactive thyroid).* https://www.mayoclinic.org/diseases-conditions/hyperthyroidism/symptoms-causes/syc-20373659

McGurgan, I. J., & Nicholl, D. J. (2017). Weber's and Rinne's tests: Bad vibrations? *Practical Neurology, 17*(4), 323–324. https://doi.org/10.1136/practneurol-2017-001611

National Center for Biotechnology Information. (2018, April 19). *How does the thyroid gland work?* https://www.ncbi.nlm.nih.gov/books/NBK279388/

Ng, S. K., Lee, D. L., Li, A. M., Wing, Y. K., & Tong, M. C. (2010). Reproducibility of clinical grading of tonsillar size. *Archives of Otolaryngology – Head & Neck Surgery, 136*(2), 159–162. https://doi.org/10.1001/archoto.2009.170

Stanford Children's Health. (n.d.). *Anatomy and physiology of the ear.* https://www.stanfordchildrens.org/en/topic/default?id=anatomy-and-physiology-of-the-ear-90-P02025

University of Washington Department of Medicine. (n.d.). *Introduction: Examination of thyroid.* https://depts.washington.edu/physdx/thyroid/index.html

Williams, E., Chillag, S., & Rizvi, A. (2014). Thyroid bruit and the underlying 'inferno.' *The American Journal of Medicine, 127*(6), 489–490.

CHAPTER 16

Assessment of the Transgender Patient

Vanessa Pomarico, EdD, APRN, FNP-BC, FAANP

 CASE STUDY

New Patient Presenting to Primary Care Office

- 34-year-old transgender male
- History of testosterone supplementation x five years

| **T** 98.9°F oral | **HR** 88 bpm | **BP** 142/98 | **RR** 12 | **O2** 99% | **Pain** 0/10 |

Max, 34 years old, presents to the office to establish care as a new patient of your practice. Max's natal sex is female, but he identifies as male. He transitioned from female to male five years ago. He has already made a social transition with his family and friends. He is currently unemployed. Max has been obtaining testosterone from the internet. He has not had any healthcare for at least the past five years.

His past medical history includes smoking one pack of cigarettes per day for 15 years and depression. He reports that he has not had any blood work drawn since college. He has NKDA and NKFA. The only medication he is taking is testosterone 100 mg IM every seven days. The remainder of his PMH is noncontributory. PSH includes eustachian tubes as a child and a tonsillectomy at age 8. He is divorced from his wife of 10 years.

Family history is significant for hypercoagulability disorder in mother, maternal aunt, and maternal first cousins. He reports his maternal grandmother died from a pulmonary embolism.

QUESTION 16.1 (Multiple choice)

Transgender is defined as:

A) A discomfort or distress that occurs as the result of an incongruity between how a person identifies and the gender assigned at birth

B) A person who is physically, romantically, and emotionally attracted toward a person regardless of their gender

C) An individual whose gender identity or gender expression differs from the sex assigned at birth

D) A person who wears clothing typically for that of the opposite sex for erotic arousal or emotional or psychological reasons

Answer: C

RATIONALE

A *transgender person* is someone whose self-identification does not align with the sex assigned at birth. Transgender persons are gender minorities who are considered to be a vulnerable population. The term *transgender* encompasses different outward expressions and gender-variant identities (Institute of Medicine, 2011). More and more people are identifying as something other than the gender binary of male or female, masculine or feminine; therefore, it is imperative that healthcare providers are educated on the appropriate terminology and self-identifying descriptions for this population of patients.

Answer A is the definition of gender dysphoria. Answer B describes someone who identifies as bisexual or pansexual. Answer D is the definition of a crossdresser. The term *transvestite* is no longer used and is considered a derogatory term.

QUESTION 16.2 (Multiple choice)

Natal sex is best defined by which of the following statements?

A) The gender or sex one is assigned at birth

B) How one identifies their gender as an adult

C) An internal sense of self

D) Deciding whether one is male or female

Answer: A

> **RATIONALE**
> *Natal sex* is the gender or sex one is born with that correlates with the corresponding reproductive organs. *Gender identity* is how one self-identifies their gender or an internal sense of self (Human Rights Campaign [HRC], 2020). *Gender binary* is based on the stereotypical male or female, masculine or feminine.

QUESTION 16.3 (True or false)
All transgender persons will have gender-affirming surgery.

Answer: False

> **RATIONALE**
> Some transgender persons desire hormone therapy and undergo gender-affirming (or gender-confirming) surgical procedures. *Gender reassignment* is a term that may pervade the literature but is no longer an appropriate term used when describing gender surgery. Some transgender persons may choose to use hormone therapy and never have any type of gender-affirming procedures. Some transgender persons may choose to identify as such and never take hormones or undergo any type of surgical procedure, while others may not even identify as transgender because they never truly accepted the gender assigned to them at birth (Coleman et al., 2022).

Some patients may elect to have surgical procedures that will create a more gender-congruent appearance. Typical surgeries for a transgender male patient include chest reconstruction or masculinizing "top surgery." This type of surgery differs in approach from a mastectomy for breast cancer to help create more natural contours of the body (Legg, 2018). Some transgender males may elect to undergo a complete hysterectomy and bilateral salpingo-oophorectomy (removal of the uterus, fallopian tubes, and ovaries; Legg, 2018). If a patient chooses to have this surgery, it is important to discuss fertility preservation such as harvesting and freezing eggs for future use. The effects of testosterone also impede the body's ability to ovulate; therefore, if a transgender male wants to consider fathering a child in the future, it is important for the healthcare provider to provide the patient with these options prior to surgery or starting testosterone therapy (Legg, 2018).

Other surgical procedures for transgender males include *metoidioplasty,* which is a less involved one-step surgery so the patient can void while standing and preserve sensitive nerve endings in the clitoris. A *total phalloplasty* is a much more labor-intensive surgery that creates a neophallus from extragenital tissue and insertion of a penile prosthesis. A *scrotoplasty* uses the labia minora and majora to create a scrotum with insertion of testicular implants (Djordjevic et al., 2019).

Transfeminine or transgender females may elect to have breast augmentation surgery. *Orchiectomy* (removal of the testes) is another gender-affirming surgery that will significantly decrease testosterone production, something that is desirable for many transgender females. Vaginoplasty is the creation of a neovagina through the use of preservation of scrotal tissue and other nerve-sparing surgery to enhance physical sensations postoperatively (Legg, 2018).

QUESTION 16.4 (Multiple choice)

Which of the following is considered not true regarding sexual orientation?

A) It is a physical attraction toward a particular gender or genders.

B) It can be toward more than one gender.

C) It is the same thing as gender identity.

D) It is a romantic attraction toward a person.

Answer: C

RATIONALE

Sexual orientation "describes sexual attraction only and is not directly related to gender identity. The sexual orientation of transgender people should be defined by the individual" (University of California, San Francisco [UCSF], 2016, para. 12). Sexual orientation is the romantic, physical, and psychological attraction toward another person (HRC, 2020). Transgender persons can be attracted to other transgender persons or *cisgender* persons (a person whose gender identity agrees with their birth gender). Whatever gender a person identifies as can be attracted to males, females, or nonbinary persons. A transgender male whose natal sex may have been female but has transitioned to male may be attracted to other males or strictly to females. Any person who is attracted to someone of the same sex is considered to be gay or lesbian. The term *homosexual* is considered an offensive term and is discouraged from use due to its derogatory nature (GLAAD, 2018).

Gender identity is best described as one's internal sense of self with respect to gender (UCSF, 2016). It is a psychological self-description or perception of being male or female, masculine or feminine. It is an awareness of belonging to a particular gender or a combination of more than one gender (HRC, n.d.-b).

QUESTION 16.5 (Multiple choice)

Considering Max's history, which of the following statements best describes his sexual orientation?

A) Heterosexual male

B) Gay male

C) Lesbian

D) Nonbinary

Answer: A

RATIONALE

Max identifies as a male and is attracted physically, romantically, and psychologically to females. He was married to a female for 10 years. Based on his self-identification as a male, he would be considered a heterosexual male—someone whose romantic, physical, and emotional attraction is toward those of the opposite sex (GLAAD, 2018). If Max were attracted to other males (cisgender or transgender males), he would identify as a gay male. Lesbians are females who are attracted to other females. Max identifies as male, so answer "C" is incorrect. Max identifies as male; therefore, answer "D" is incorrect because *nonbinary* refers to someone who identifies as neither male nor female and is not related to sexual orientation.

QUESTION 16.6 (Multiple choice)

Which of the following statements correctly describes a person who is pangender?

A) A woman who is attracted to other women

B) A person who is attracted to a person regardless of that person's gender identity, gender description, or sexual orientation

C) A person whose gender presentation or gender variation differs from the societal norm

D) A person who is attracted to both men and women

Answer: C

RATIONALE

The correct answer, C, is the only answer that describes gender identity. Answers A, B, and D are descriptions of sexual orientation and not gender identity.

It is important for nurses and healthcare providers to know the differences between *sexual orientation* (who a person is attracted to emotionally, sexually, and physically); *gender identity* (how one perceives and recognizes their own gender); and *nonbinary gender* (identifying as neither male nor female, masculine nor feminine; National Center for Transgender Equality, 2023). Table 16.1 lists some of this terminology.

TABLE 16.1 Culturally Sensitive Gender-Identity and Sexual-Orientation Terminology

Sexual Orientation	Gender Identity	Nonbinary Gender
Straight	Cisgender	Agender
Gay	Transgender male	Androgyne
Lesbian	Transgender female	Bigender
Bisexual	Gender-neutral	Nonbinary
Pansexual	Two-spirit	Queer
Queer		Gender-fluid
Asexual		Gender variant
		Pangender
		Third gender

Sexual Orientation

Sexual orientation is not related to gender identity and simply describes one's sexual attraction to a person (UCSF, 2016). The term *straight* refers to a person who is heterosexual and is attracted to members of the opposite sex. *Gay* describes a male who is attracted to other males. *Lesbian* refers to a female who is attracted to other females. *Bisexual* is a term that describes a person who is attracted to more than one sex or gender (HRC, n.d.-b). A person who identifies as *pansexual* is attracted to other persons regardless of their own gender identity, gender description, or sexual orientation (Moradini et al., 2017).

Gender Identity

A person whose gender identity and gender expression align with their sex assigned at birth is *cisgender* (Fenway Institute, 2020). A *transgender male* is a person whose natal sex is female but identifies as male. A *transgender female* is a person whose natal sex is male but identifies as a female. *Gender fluid* refers to a person who does not have one fixed gender (Baker, 2018).

A person who identifies as *pangender* (also referred to as *bigender* or *polygender*) is one whose gender variations are different from that of the societal norm or gender binary (Fenway Institute, 2020). *Third gender* and *two-spirit* are terms that describe a person who has characteristic traits of both men and women. These terms are a derivative of native North American cultures (Indian Health Service, 2019).

Nonbinary

Nonbinary persons do not identify as any one particular gender, male or female (UCSF, 2016). Persons who identify as *agender* consider themselves identifying without a particular fixed gender. The term *androgyne* is used by those who may identify as both male and female or neither male nor female. They may present ambiguously and choose to take on an ambiguous name (Fenway Institute, 2020). *Bigender* is also used interchangeably with the term *pangender*. The term *queer* at one time was considered derogatory and still is if used in the incorrect context. For example, stating "That person is so queer" is derogatory, versus "They identify as queer," which is acceptable if that is the term with which someone identifies. *Queer* describes those persons who have a nonbinary gender identity.

Gender Pronouns or Gender-Neutral Pronouns

The English language does not have a gender-neutral pronoun, but it is important for nurses to recognize the differences in the use of preferred pronouns when caring for a transgender patient. Table 16.2 lists some of the more common preferred gender pronouns. Typically, third-person plural pronouns describe a group of people, and commonly it is not considered grammatically correct to use third-person plural when referring to one. However, there are many people who identify their gender or lack of gender identification by using third-person pronouns (Trans Student Educational Resources, 2019). It is now accepted as grammatically correct to do so (Baron, n.d.).

TABLE 16.2 Gender Pronouns or Gender-Neutral Pronouns

Subjective	Objective	Possessive
He	Him	His
She	Her	Hers
They	Them	Theirs
Ze/Zi	Zer/Zir	Zers/Zirs

QUESTION 16.7 (Multiple choice)

The provider is unsure how to address Max. Which of the following statements is correct?

A) "What is your preferred pronoun?"

B) "Do you prefer that I call you Mister or Miss?"

C) "What is the name on your birth certificate?"

D) "Have you legally changed your name?"

Answer: A

RATIONALE

Asking a patient their chosen name and their pronoun demonstrates the provider's acceptance and knowledge in using appropriate and correct terminology. Answer B demonstrates gender binary and completely excludes any person who does not identify as masculine or feminine. Answers C and D are both incorrect because transgender patients may not have had their birth certificates amended or changed their names legally, often a costly endeavor. Also, if patients change their gender markers and need future surgery on the reproductive organs they were born with, insurance may not cover these procedures if the patient has legally changed their gender markers.

A transgender person may be hesitant to reveal their natal sex or gender due to fear of discrimination. Many transgender persons have prior negative experiences with healthcare providers or have been harassed or experienced acts of violence—and therefore have a fear of being stigmatized or denied healthcare (Buttaro et al., 2017). A survey done by the National LGBTQ Task Force revealed that 33% of respondents who saw a provider during the previous year had a negative experience, were denied or refused care, or had to teach the provider about transgender people to receive care (James et al., 2016).

QUESTION 16.8 (Multiple choice)

Which of the following would be the most worrisome in a person who is taking testosterone?

A) Acne

B) Hirsutism

C) Abnormal liver function tests

D) Unilateral lower extremity pain and swelling

Answer: D

RATIONALE

The use of testosterone may increase the risk of acne, but this can easily be treated with topical or oral antibiotics. Hirsutism is a desired effect of testosterone therapy, especially in transgender males. Testosterone is metabolized in the liver. Assessing liver function is important to determine any abnormal liver function as a result of testosterone therapy, and a serum testosterone level will demonstrate the effectiveness of testosterone therapy. Max has been obtaining testosterone from an unknown source. Many transgender persons without health insurance will obtain testosterone via the internet or black market. The purity of these products in unknown, and they can contain fillers that further dilute the inert ingredient.

A Doppler would be indicated if the patient was complaining of unilateral leg pain and swelling to rule out deep vein thrombosis (DVT). People who take testosterone are at a higher risk for developing a DVT due to polycythemia or erythrocytosis that can occur as a result of testosterone therapy. It is important to check CBC/diff to rule out erythrocytosis. *Erythrocytosis* or *polycythemia* is an increase in hemoglobin, hematocrit, and red blood cell counts causing an increased risk for development of a DVT. Max's BMI is classified as morbidly obese. He smokes one pack of cigarettes per day and has a history of hypercoagulability disorder in his family, all of which places him at greater risk for developing a DVT (Mayo Clinic, 2022).

QUESTION 16.9 (Multiple response)

Max recently started a new job. On the first day, he avoided using the restroom due to concerns for his safety. It would be important to discuss which of the following with Max prior to his employment: *(Select all that apply)*

A) Inquire about gender-neutral restrooms in the workplace.

B) A social transition through human resources reminding employees of the protocols in place against any discrimination toward any transgender person.

C) Giving Max a key to the private restroom.

D) Educating Max on the risk of developing a urinary tract infection (UTI) due to holding his urine for too long.

E) Assess Max's risk factors and support system.

Answer: A, B, D, E

RATIONALE

It is important for Max to discuss with his new employer his concerns of being transgender and his safety as part of the Equal Employment Opportunity Commission onboarding information. Although many transgender persons do not want people to know about their transition, many of them must alert their employers due to insurance concerns (HRC, n.d.-a). Max identifies as male, but since he still has female reproductive anatomy, he is still female on his insurance. Max presents as male, but if his physical appearance does not correlate with that of the societal norm of a typical male, Max could be placed in harm's way by using the traditional male restroom. Human resources should review their protocols with employees regarding discrimination prior to Max starting work. It is of vital importance to discuss with Max the risk of UTI development and urinary retention, as well as ascertaining who his support system is outside of the workplace. Answer C is incorrect because having his own key to a private restroom will just perpetuate any discrimination and could further cause speculation by other employees.

QUESTION 16.10 **(Multiple response)**

Max reports his fear of dating again. He states that his wife left him "broken-hearted on many levels." He shares that his wife became angry when he decided to transition and reportedly told him that she was no longer attracted to him because she was a lesbian and was only attracted to other women. Which of the following are considered to be abusive acts? *(Select all that apply)*

A) Berating Max in front of others

B) Withholding affection

C) Running up credit card debt

D) Accusing Max of neglect

E) Abuse only occurs in males.

Answer: A, B, C

RATIONALE

Intimate partner violence (IPV) is a form of abuse that can present in many different forms: physically, emotionally, financially, and sexually (World Health Organization, 2012). In the LGBTQIA+ community, abuse can also present when a person tries to "out" their partner socially when the person is not ready to reveal this information to others. It can also occur among the LGBTQIA+ community when someone denies a person's gender identity, intentionally misgenders them, denies access to hormones, rejects the person socially or in front of others as a means to turn others against them, and controls the finances, especially if one is unemployed at the time. It is a myth that abuse only occurs in males (Brown & Herman, 2015).

The National Intimate Partner and Sexual Violence Survey maintains the most current local and national data on IPV, victimization, and sexual assault in the United States (Centers for Disease Control and Prevention, n.d.). Safety, outing themselves through disclosure, community attitudes toward transgender persons, gender stereotypes, and transphobia are among some of the many concerns for transgender persons (Henry et al., 2018). This also includes people who do not use appropriate and gender-affirming terminology, misgendering the person by intentionally using the wrong gender descriptors, bullying, and harassment. Crossing physical and emotional boundaries through touching, physical abuse, and acts of violence are higher in this population. Data on IPV among transgender persons is truly deficient (Health Resources & Services Administration, 2017). It is critical for nurses and all healthcare providers to be aware of available screening surveys and resources for patients who are at risk for IPV.

The National Transgender Discrimination Survey, conducted in 2015 (James et al., 2016), revealed that 90% of the respondents reported being mistreated, harassed, or discriminated against at their place of employment. Additionally, 47% were denied promotion, fired, or were not hired. The vast majority of the respondents (71%) attempted to conceal their gender and transition in an attempt to avoid any harassment or violent acts against them. Transgender persons endure double the rate of unemployment in the US (14% versus 7% of the general population).

The rate of suicide among transgender persons is a staggering 41% versus the national average of 1.6% (James et al., 2016). Transgender persons of color have experienced the highest rate of discrimination and sexual and physical assault against them. In an effort to survive economically, some transgender persons who are unable to secure employment or have been fired will often turn to sex work, selling drugs, or other underground work (James et al., 2016). Transgender persons also more frequently experience violent acts during imprisonment, including physical and sexual assault.

Nurses are the best advocates for their patients and are in the best position to identify at-risk patients, especially transgender persons. Understanding the unique needs of this population, learning the correct terminology, and connecting the patient with the appropriate resources will go a long way in the health and well-being of transgender persons. Should a patient disclose mistreatment or abuse, some appropriate responses might include (Basham et al., 2019, PPT slide 17):

- "Thank you for telling me."
- "I'm sorry this is happening."
- "You do not deserve this."
- "You are not alone."
- "We can help."

QUESTION 16.11 (Short answer)
Considering Max's assessment and disclosures during this exam, what are three nursing priorities for his care?

1. _____

2. _____

3. _____

ANSWER(S)/RATIONALE

Considering Max's clinical presentation and history, nursing priorities for his care might include:

- Screening for anxiety, depression, or suicidal ideation: Max has an established history of depression based on his subjective history. He has been under a lot of stress with his recent divorce.

- Screening for IPV: Max reveals during the visit that his ex-wife displayed abusive tendencies. Even though the marriage has ended, the nurse can screen for IPV to assure the patient is not involved in an unsafe relationship.

- Administration of safety assessments and referral to appropriate agencies for service and refuge: Screening for home safety and safe routine activities helps the nurse identify if the patient is at an additional risk or may need referral for social services.

- Physical assessment for adverse reactions to hormone replacement: Max is receiving testosterone therapy; monitoring for adverse effects is necessary for patient safety and should be reported to the prescriber if identified.

- Patient education on sexually transmitted diseases: Max is considering re-entering the dating scene. Patient education on safe sex practices may reduce the likelihood of sexually transmitted infection.

- Patient education on smoking cessation: The patient revealed in his subjective history that he has been a smoker for over 15 years. Smoking cigarettes is associated with many comorbid health conditions.

- Patient education on healthy eating and risks associated with obesity: The calculated BMI for this patient is 49.56, which is classified as morbidly obese.

CHAPTER 16 WORKSHEET

Based on my initial assessment, I thought:

_____

_____

_____

Based on my revised/informed assessment, I now know:

_____

_____

_____

A nursing priority for this patient would be _____

because _____

After completing this chapter, something I have learned is:

_____

_____

_____

After completing this chapter, something I need more clarity on is:

_____

_____

_____

After completing this chapter, something else I want to learn is:

_____

_____

_____

REFERENCES

Baker, W. B. (2018). Sexual and gender identities in transgender men: Fluid and binary perspectives. *Journal of Gay & Lesbian Mental Health, 22*(3), 280–301. https://doi.org/10.1080/19359705.2018.1458677

Baron, D. (n.d.). A brief history of singular 'they.' *Oxford English Dictionary.* https://www.oed.com/discover/a-brief-history-of-singular-they/?tl=true

Basham, C., Presley, C., & Potter, J. (2019). *Implementing routine intimate partner violence screening in a primary care setting.* https://www.lgbthealtheducation.org/wp-content/uploads/Screening-for-IPV-in-Primary-Care-Webinar.pdf

Brown, T. N., & Herman, J. L. (2015). *Intimate partner violence and sexual abuse among LGBT people: A review of existing literature.* The Williams Institute. https://williamsinstitute.law.ucla.edu/publications/ipv-sex-abuse-lgbt-people/

Buttaro, T., Trybulski, J., Polgar-Bailey, P., & Sandberg-Cook, J. (2017). *Primary care: A collaborative practice* (5th ed.). Elsevier.

Centers for Disease Control and Prevention. (n.d.). *National Intimate Partner and Sexual Violence Survey (NISVS).* https://www.cdc.gov/violenceprevention/datasources/nisvs/index.html

Coleman, E., Radix, A. E., Bouman, W. P., Brown, G. R., de Vries, A. L. C., Deutsch, M. B., Ettner, R., Fraser, L, Goodman, M., Green, J., Hancock, A. B., Johnson, T. W., Karasic, D. H., Knudson, G. A., Leibowitz, S. F., Meyer-Bahlburg, H. F., L., Monstrey, S. J., Motmans, J., Nahata, L., Nieder, T. O., Reisner, S. L., Richards, C., Schechter, L. S., Tangpricha, V., Tishelman, A. C., Van Trotsenburg, M. A. A., Winter, S., Ducheny, K., Adams, N. J., Adrián, T. M., Allen, L. R., Azul, D., Bagga, H., Başar, K., Bathory, D. S., Belinky, J. J., Berg, D. R., Berli, J. U., Bluebond-Langner, R. O., Bouman, M.-B., Bowers, M. L., Brassard, P. J., Byrne, J., Capitán, L., Cargill, C. J., Carswell, J. M., Chang, S. C., Chelvakumar, G., Corneil, T., Dalke, K. B., De Cuypere, G., de Vries, E., Den Heijer, M., Devor, A. H., Dhejne, C., D'Marco, A., Edmiston, E. K., Edwards-Leeper, L., Ehrbar, R., Ehrensaft, D., Eisfeld, J., Elaut, E., Erickson-Schroth, L., Feldman, J. L., Fisher, A. D., Garcia, M. M., Gijs, L., Green, S. E., Hall, B. P., Hardy, T. L. D., Irwig, M. S., Jacobs, L. A., Janssen, A. C., Johnson, K., Klink, D. T., Kreukels, B. P. C., Kuper, L. E., Kvach, E. J., Malouf, M. A., Massey, R., Mazur, T., McLachlan, C., Morrison, S. D., Mosser, S. W., Neira, P. M., Nygren, U., Oates, J. M., Obedin-Maliver, J., Pagkalos, G., Patton, J., Phanuphak, N., Rachlin, K., Reed, T., Rider, G. N., Ristori, J., Robbins-Cherry, S., Roberts, S. A., Rodriguez-Wallberg, K. A., Rosenthal, S. M., Sabir, K., Safer, J. D., Scheim, A. I., Seal, L. J., Sehoole, T. J., Spencer, K., St. Amand, C., Steensma, T. D., Strang, J. F., Taylor, G. B., Tilleman, K., T'Sjoen, G. G., Vala, L. N., Van Mello, N. M., Veale, J. F., Vencill, J. A., Vincent, B., Wesp, L. M., West, M. A., & Arcelus, J. (2022). Standards of care for the health of transgender and gender diverse people, version 8. *International Journal of Transgender Health, 23*(Suppl. 1), S1–259. https://doi.org/10.1080/26895269.2022.2100644

Djordjevic, M. L., Stojanovic, B., & Bizic, M. (2019). Metoidioplasty: Techniques and outcomes. *Translational Andrology and Urology, 8*(3), 248–253. https://doi.org/10.21037/tau.2019.06.12

Fenway Institute. (2020). *LGBTQIA+ glossary of terms for health care teams.* https://www.lgbtqiahealtheducation.org/publication/lgbtqia-glossary-of-terms-for-health-care-teams/

GLAAD. (2018). *GLAAD media reference guide* (11th ed.). https://glaad.org/reference/trans-terms/

Health Resources & Services Administration. (2017). *The HRSA strategy to address intimate partner violence 2017–2020.* https://www.hrsa.gov/sites/default/files/hrsa/HRSA-strategy-intimate-partner-violence.pdf

Henry, R. S., Perrin, P. B., Coston, B. M., & Calton, J. M. (2018). Intimate partner violence and mental health among transgender/gender nonconforming adults. *Journal of Interpersonal Violence, 36*(7–8). https://doi.org/10.1177/0886260518775148

Human Rights Campaign. (n.d.-a). *Coming out at work*. https://www.hrc.org/resources/coming-out-at-work

Human Rights Campaign. (n.d.-b). *Sexual orientation and gender identity definitions*. https://www.hrc.org/resources/sexual-orientation-and-gender-identity-terminology-and-definitions

Indian Health Service. (2019). *Lesbian, gay, bisexual, transgender, questioning (LGBTQ), and two-spirit health*. https://www.ihs.gov/lgbt/health/twospirit/

Institute of Medicine. (2011). *The health of lesbian, gay, bisexual, and transgender people: Building a foundation for better understanding*. National Academies Press.

James, S. E., Herman, J. L., Rankin, S., Keisling, M., Mottet, L., & Anafi, M. (2016). *The report of the 2015 US Transgender Survey*. National Center for Transgender Equality. https://Transequality.org/sites/default/files/docs/usts/USTS-Full-Report-Dec17.pdf

Legg, T. J. (2018). *What to expect from gender confirmation surgery*. https://www.healthline.com/health/transgender/gender-confirmation-surgery

Mayo Clinic. (2022). *Deep vein thrombosis (DVT)*. https://www.mayoclinic.org/diseases-conditions/deep-vein-thrombosis/symptoms-causes/syc-20352557

Morandini, J. S., Blaszczynski, A., & Dar-Nimrod, I. (2017). Who adopts queer and pansexual sexual identities? *Journal of Sex Research, 54*(7), 911–922. https://doi.org/10.1080/00224499.2016.1249332

National Center for Transgender Equality. (2023). *Understanding nonbinary people: How to be respectful and supportive*. https://transequality.org/issues/resources/understanding-non-binary-people-how-to-be-respectful-and-supportive

Trans Student Educational Resources. (2019). *Gender pronouns*. http://www.transstudent.org/pronouns101

University of California, San Francisco. (2016). *Transgender care: Terminology and definitions*. https://transcare.ucsf.edu/guidelines/terminology

University of Wisconsin, Milwaukee. (2019). *Gender pronouns*. https://uwm.edu/lgbtrc/support/gender-pronouns/

World Health Organization. (2012). *Intimate partner violence*. https://apps.who.int/iris/bitstream/handle/10665/77432/WHO_RHR_12.36_eng.pdf;jsessionid=7FDAC7B3E410AD039AFB08174261D424?sequence=1

Practice Test

1. When assessing a patient's level of consciousness using the Glasgow Coma Scale (GCS), the nurse interprets a score of 4 as:

   A) Normal function   C) Moderate brain injury

   B) Minor brain injury   D) Severe brain injury

2. At the change of shift, the nurse reads the narrative note from the previous shift. The patient is noted to have miotic pupils, meaning:

   A) Dilated   C) Uneven

   B) Constricted   D) Unreactive

3. A 60-year-old client recently suffered a hemorrhagic stroke. Following the stroke, his family reports changes to his affect and personality. This is most likely the result of damage to:

   A) Frontal lobe   C) Broca's area

   B) Pariteal lobe   D) Occipital lobe

4. The nurse is performing a focused neurological assessment for a patient with optic migraines. He proceeds to examine the patient's extraocular motion by performing the six cardinal fields of gaze test. What cranial nerves are being tested during this exam?

   A) 3, 4, 6   C) 3, 6, 7

   B) 5, 7, 8   D) 2, 5, 8

5. During a neurological exam, the patient is unable to correctly identify the smell of cinnamon. This may potentially indicate an issue with cranial nerve _____.

   A) 3   C) 4

   B) 2   D) 1

6. The nurse auscultates a new onset murmur in a 22-year-old male. The murmur occurs between S2 and the subsequent S1. This would be classified as a:

   A) Systolic murmur   **C)** Benign murmur

   B) Diastolic murmur   **D)** Pathological murmur

7. Which of the following statements is *true* regarding the correct stethoscope placement during cardiac auscultation?

   A) The aortic valve can be auscultated at the 2nd intercostal space at the left sternal border.

   B) Erb's point can be auscultated at the 3rd intercostal space at the left sternal border.

   C) The pulmonic valve can be auscultated at the 4th intercostal space at the right sternal border.

   D) The tricuspid valve can be auscultated at the 5th intercostal space at the midclavicular line.

8. When examining the neck, the nurse appreciates a prominent bulging of the jugular vein. This condition may indicate fluid volume overload and is known as:

   A) Carotid bruit   **C)** Jugular venous distention

   B) Thyroidmegaly   **D)** Tracheal deviation

9. You are assessing your patient diagnosed with exacerbated congestive heart failure (CHF). Which abnormal heart sound is correlated with systemic volume overload in CHF?

   A) S_3 **C)** Mitral click

   B) Split S_1 **D)** S_2

10. The nurse is documenting vital signs from morning rounds. He records the patient's pulse as "regular, 72 bpm, 3+". This means:

    A) The pulse was regular in occurrence at a rate of 72 and is bounding in strength.

    B) The pulse was irregular in occurrence at a rate of 72 and is thready in strength.

    C) The pulse was regular in occurrence at a rate of 72 and is normal in strength.

    D) The pulse was irregular in occurrence at a rate of 72 and is diminished in strength.

11. A patient with a history of hyperlipidemia and hypertension presents to his primary care provider with complaints of leg pain that occurs when walking and dissipates at rest. He is concerned because his father had a similar condition that was related to arterial blockage in the legs. This leg pain is known as:

    A) Deep vein thrombosis   C) Intermittent claudication

    B) Varicose veins   D) Terminal ischemia

12. As the nurse proceeds with an examination of the skin, hair, and nails, he notices the capillary refill to be six seconds. This is significant because:

    A) It is a normal capillary refill.

    B) This indicates brisk refill, which indicates good circulation.

    C) This indicates sluggish refill, which indicates poor circulation.

    D) This indicates brisk refill, which indicates adequate hydration.

13. A patient presents with complaints of nausea, vomiting, and diarrhea for the past three days. She has not been able to tolerate food or fluids. The nurse is concerned about the patient's hydration status. Which of the following exam techniques would indicate the patient's hydration status?

    A) Capillary refill   C) Schamroth's sign

    B) Murphy's sign   D) Skin turgor

14. When evaluating a skin lesion for potential malignancy, the nurse recognizes that a lesion greater than _____ in diameter is considered to be highly suspicious.

    A) 6 mm   C) 4 mm

    B) 5 mm   D) 3 mm

15. After performing an assessment of the skin, the nurse proceeds to document his findings. During the examination, he noticed a single, flat, hyperpigmented lesion with symmetric borders and a diameter of 5 mm. The nurse would document this lesion as a:

    A) Papule   C) Vesicle

    B) Macule   D) Patch

16. A nurse working in a long-term care facility is taking care of a 75-year-old female patient. The patient tells the nurse she is concerned about the dark spots she has noticed on the back of her hands. The nurse tells the patient that these spots likely represent:

    A) Melanoma   C) Senile purpura

    B) Pediculus humanus   D) Tinea corporis

17. Which symptoms may indicate that a patient with hypothyroidism may require an increase in their thyroid replacement medication? *(Select all that apply)*

    A) Fatigue   D) Cold intolerance

    B) Bulging eyes   E) Weight gain

    C) Hair loss

18. While examining the left tympanic membrane, the nurse appreciates the tympanic reflection, known as the cone of light, at:

    A) 3 o'clock   C) 7 o'clock

    B) 5 o'clock   D) 9 o'clock

19. An 18-month old boy presents with his mother, who suspects her son has an ear infection. He had been up all night with a low-grade fever and has been tugging at his right ear lobe. When proceeding with the otoscopic exam, the nurse correctly positions the ear lobe by:

    A) Pulling the helix up and back

    B) Compressing the tragus

    C) Pushing down on the lobule

    D) Pulling the helix down and out

20. While assessing a patient's lymph nodes, the nurse notes a tender, mobile lymph node palpable directly in front of the ear. When documenting the lymphadenopathy, the nurse documents tenderness of the _____ nodes.

    A) Submental   C) Jugulodigastric

    B) Preauricular   D) Superficial cervical

21. A patient diagnosed with streptococcal pharyngitis is observed to have tonsils with patchy exudate occupying approximately 60% of the oropharyngeal width. The tonsils are graded as:

    A) 1+   C) 3+
    B) 2+   D) 4+

22. Your patient was diagnosed with acute cholecystitis. As the nurse assigned to this patient, you understand that the patient will most likely have the following symptom:

    A) Epigastric pain that is relieved with eating
    B) Epigastric pain that is aggravated with a high fat meal
    C) Left lower quadrant with rebound tenderness
    D) A negative Murphy's sign

23. You are educating a patient who has been diagnosed with cirrhosis about esophageal varices. You advise the patient to avoid the following activities, if possible: *(Select all that apply)*

    A) Consuming alcohol
    B) Vomiting
    C) Sleeping in a lateral recumbent position
    D) Eating spicy foods
    E) Excessive coughing

24. Your patient was recently admitted with acute pancreatitis. As the nurse caring for this patient, you know the patient's risk factors include all *except*:

    A) Heavy alcohol use   C) Diabetes mellitus
    B) Smoking   D) Obesity

25. A patient is admitted to the ED with complaint of pain around the umbilicus that radiates to the lower abdominal region on the right. Pain is elicited while palpating the right lower quadrant of the abdomen (about one-third the distance between the anterior superior iliac spine and the umbilicus). This is known as:

    A) Positive Murphy's sign   C) Positive McBurney's sign
    B) Positive Rovsing's sign   D) Positive Trousseau's sign

26. You are the nurse taking care of a patient that is four days post-op after an appendectomy. Which assessment finding requires further evaluation?

    A) The patient reports only tolerating clear liquids.

    B) The patient reports incisional pain.

    C) The patient reports his last bowel movement was pre-operative.

    D) A and C

27. You are providing education to a patient newly diagnosed with a duodenal ulcer. Which of the following statements indicates that reeducation may be needed?

    A) "I should eat smaller meals throughout the day instead of three large ones."

    B) "I should avoid coffee, chocolate, and fried foods."

    C) "Eating will only make my pain worse."

    D) "I should report any dark, tarry bowel movements."

28. You are caring for a patient who presented to the hospital with a temperature of 101.9°F and abdominal pain. Workup in the emergency department included sending blood samples to the lab for a variety of tests. A complete blood count revealed an elevated white blood cell count. It is suspected that your patient has diverticulitis. Which of the following statements is correct regarding diverticulitis?

    A) Oatmeal and nuts are the best foods for acute diverticulitis.

    B) Diverticulitis is usually associated with a positive Cullen's sign.

    C) Patients with diverticulitis should be encouraged to drink clear liquids.

    D) A positive Murphy's sign is indicative of diverticulitis.

29. The nurse is performing an obstetrical history and needs the date of the last menstrual period to determine the estimated date of birth using Nagel's rule. The nurse asks the patient:

    A) What was the last day of your last period?

    B) What was the heaviest day of your last menstrual period?

    C) What was the first day of your last menstrual cycle?

    D) What was the last month you had a menstrual period?

30. The patient presents with complaints of frequent urge to void, nausea and vomiting, burning during urination, chills, fever, costal vertebral angle tenderness, and pain in the lower abdomen radiating to the back. The nurse correctly suspects the following condition:

    A) Cystitis

    B) Pregnancy

    C) Ovarian cyst

    D) Pyelonephritis

31. During patient teaching, the nurse explains gynecological care and steps to take to prevent sexually transmitted infections (STIs). *(Select all that apply)*

    A) Limit the number of sexual partners.

    B) Get tested yearly for chlamydia and gonorrhea after 25 years of age.

    C) Use condoms consistently.

    D) Talk to your sexual partners about their history with STI.

    E) Ask your provider if STI screening is offered.

32. The patient presents to the ED and explains she is currently pregnant, has a 3-year-old child born at 39 weeks, and also lost a pregnancy in the first trimester. The nurse documents her GTPAL as:

    A) G2 T1 P1 A0 L1

    B) G3 T1 P0 A1 L1

    C) G2 T0 P0 A1 L2

    D) G3 T1 P1 A0 L2

33. The nurse admits a patient into labor and delivery and needs to calculate her due date. Using Nagel's rule and the date of July 20, 2023, determine her estimated date of birth.

    A) April 27, 2024

    B) February 23, 2024

    C) March 20, 2024

    D) May 27, 2024

34. The nurse is planning a patient education program about urinary tract infections (UTIs) across the life span. Which of the following correct statements will the nurse include in the educational discussion? *(Select all that apply)*

    A) UTIs are a very common type of infection, mostly affecting children under the age of 5 and men and women aged 70 and older.

    B) People with high blood glucose levels are especially susceptible to getting a UTI.

    C) For prevention, drink plenty of water, urinate often, keep your genital area clean, and empty your bladder before and after sex.

    D) There is conclusive evidence to using cranberry supplement products to prevent UTIs.

35. The nurse in a urology practice discusses bladder health with her many patients. Which of the following female patient statements is a reason for concern? *(Select all that apply)*

    A) "I have been doing my Kegel exercises three times a day for the past two weeks, and I still do not see any improvement."

    B) "I am drinking about 2 liters of fluid a day and urinating about 500 liters."

    C) "I don't like to sit while I void, and I find myself going to the bathroom about 14 times a day."

    D) "I wipe from front to back after using the toilet."

36. When assessing the geriatric client, the nurse correctly acknowledges which of the following as a normal variant of aging?

    A) Low-frequency hearing loss

    B) Hypertrophied skin surfaces

    C) Increased muscle mass

    D) Decreased metabolism

37. A 70-year-old male presents for a wellness visit. Which of the following is expected to be included as part of routine health maintenance for this patient?

    A) Prostate specific antigen (PSA)

    B) Brain magnetic resonance imaging (MRI)

    C) Cardiac stress test

    D) BRACA-1 testing

38. Which of the following physiological changes in the elderly patient is *not* considered to be a risk factor for increased fall risk?

    A) Decreased muscle strength   C) Decreased step height

    B) Increased reflexes   D) Increased postural sway

39. When evaluating the fall risk for a patient, which tool is used to determine the patient's likelihood of falling?

    A) Downton Fall Risk Index

    B) Hendrich II Fall Risk Model

    C) Timed Up and Go test

    D) A combined assessment approach is preferred.

40. The nurse is discussing risk factors for dementia with a patient and his caregiver. When discussing potential risk factors for the development of dementia, the nurse includes: *(Select all that apply)*

    A) Obesity

    B) Decreased HDL cholesterol

    C) Hypotension

    D) Smoking

    E) Low physical exercise

41. A nurse is caring for a patient who complains of feeling short of breath. Respiratory rate is recorded at 28 breaths per minute. Before contacting the provider, the nurse should *first*:

    A) Raise the head of the bed 45 degrees

    B) Administer 2L O2 via nasal cannula

    C) Administer CPR

    D) Check the patient's blood pressure

42. A nurse is providing discharge information for a patient with recently diagnosed asthma. Which of the following common triggers for asthma should the nurse instruct the patient to try to avoid? *(Select all that apply)*

    A) Cat and dog dander

    B) Humidified rooms

    C) Sunlight

    D) Tobacco smoke

    E) Chewing tobacco

    F) Wood burning stoves

43. An African-American patient with COPD seeks emergency care for acute respiratory distress. For patients with dark skin color, the nurse should assess for cyanosis by inspecting the:

    A) Lips

    B) Mucous membranes

    C) Thorax

    D) Nail beds

44. A pediatric patient was noted to have retractions below the xyphoid process on the upper abdomen. When recording this, the nurse labels these as:

    A) Substernal retractions

    B) Subcostal retractions

    C) Intercostal retractions

    D) Supraclavicular retractions

45. A nurse is caring for an elderly patient who is suffering from influenza. The nurse performs frequent respiratory assessments, as the nurse knows that _____ is one of the most common complications of influenza.

    A) Pulmonary embolism
    B) Bacteremia
    C) Pneumonia
    D) Guillain-Barré syndrome

46. Which of the following statements best describes sexual orientation?

    A) How one identifies internally with regards to their gender
    B) The romantic, physical, and psychological attraction towards another person
    C) A person or persons who identify without a particular fixed gender
    D) The incongruence between the sex assigned at birth and how one identifies their gender

47. Which patients should the nurse ask to identify their pronouns?

    A) Patients who appear to be nonbinary
    B) Patients who self-identify as transgender
    C) Patients who identify as lesbian or gay
    D) All patients should be asked what their self-identified pronoun is.

48. Transgender patients who take hormones such as testosterone or estrogen should be monitored for the risk of developing which of the following? *(Select all that apply)*

    A) Deep vein thrombosis
    B) Hypertension
    C) Type 2 diabetes
    D) Abnormal liver function
    E) Migraines

49. Transgender persons are at higher risk for which of the following? *(Select all that apply)*

    A) Double the rate of unemployment
    B) Higher rates of death by suicide
    C) Higher socioeconomic status
    D) Acts of physical, sexual, and emotional harassment
    E) Substance abuse

50. When caring for a transgender patient, which of the following would be appropriate for the nurse to consider? *(Select all that apply)*

    A) Continuity of care by the same nurses as much as possible
    B) Educating all caregivers on the appropriate and sensitive care of the transgender patient
    C) Asking the patient to teach them about what it is like to be transgender
    D) Minimizing the patient's visitors during their hospitalization
    E) Requesting that all caregivers call the patient by their preferred pronoun

ANSWER KEY

1. D	14. A	27. C	40. A, D, E
2. B	15. B	28. C	41. A
3. A	16. C	29. C	42. A, B, D, F
4. A	17. A, D, E	30. D	43. B
5. D	18. C	31. A, C, D, E	44. A
6. B	19. D	32. B	45. C
7. B	20. B	33. A	46. B
8. C	21. C	34. A, B, C	47. D
9. A	22. B	35. B, C	48. A, B, D
10. A	23. A, B, E	36. D	49. A, B, D, E
11. C	24. C	37. A	50. A, B, E
12. C	25. B	38. B	
13. D	26. D	39. D	

NCLEX Next
Generation Questions

1. Exhibit item

Mr. Blake is an 80-year-old patient who presents status post-fall. He is awake with a contusion noted on the right elbow with no active bleeding. His past medical history is significant for hypertension.

He lives with his wife and dog. He completed high school and worked as a contractor before retiring at 65.

Vital signs: BP 118/70; HR 78; O2 saturation 96%; RR 18; SLUMS 14

When reviewing Mr. Blake's intake note, which item does the nurse recognize requires follow-up?

A) SLUMS 14

B) HR 78

C) Contusion right elbow

D) O2 saturation 96%

Answer/Rationale: A

A SLUMS score of 14 in those who completed high school likely indicates dementia. Further evaluation will be required to determine the patient's mental status, as it may increase his risk for future falls. An HR of 78 and O2 saturation of 96% are within normal limits. A nonbleeding contusion of the elbow may require further observation but is not the priority.

2. Exhibit

Hailey, who is 8 years old, presents for her annual physical. Today, she weighs 70 pounds and measures 53 inches. Use the growth chart to determine her weight-percentile.

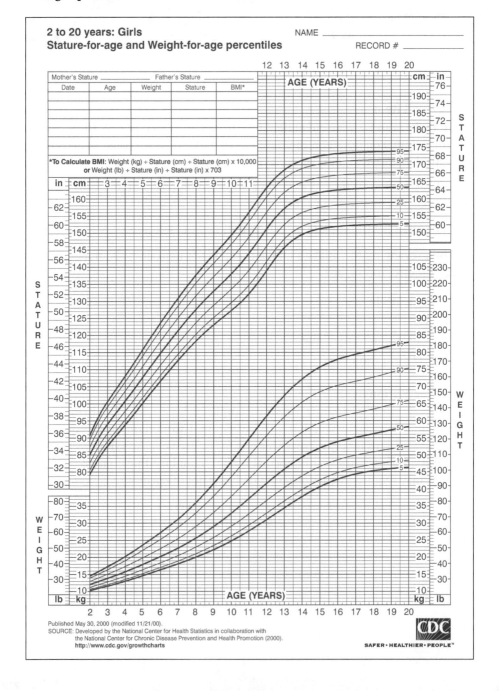

A) 90th percentile

B) 75th percentile

C) 50th percentile

D) 30th percentile

Answer/Rationale: A

The patient's gender, age, and weight place her in the 90th percentile.

3. Hot spot

A patient who has recently experienced a stroke is having difficulty with coordination. Select the area of the brain that has most likely been affected. *Place an 'x' on the image in the correct location.*

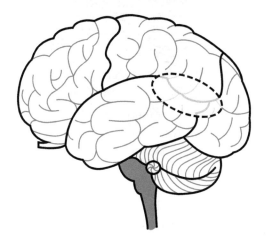

Answer/Rationale:

The cerebellum, located at the base of the brain, is responsible for coordination.

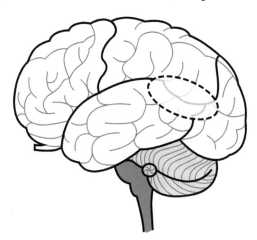

4. Hot spot

When assessing a patient with suspect left ventricular enlargement, the nurse palpates for the position of the point of maximal impulse (PMI). Where does the nurse place their fingers to palpate the PMI? *Place an 'x' on the image in the correct location.*

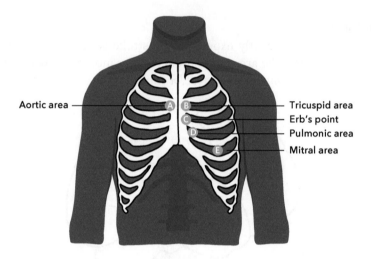

Answer/Rationale:

The PMI can be felt in the same location as mitral auscultation, the 5th/6th intercostal space at the left midclavicular line.

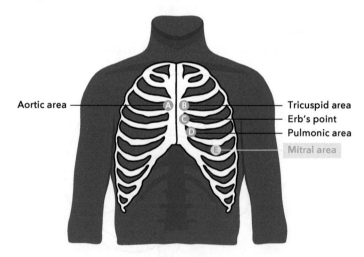

5. Matrix

A 65-year-old patient with a history of chronic bronchitis for 15 years presents to the emergency department for evaluation. When performing the physical assessment, which findings does the nurse expect to find? *Place an 'x' in the correlating box to indicate if the finding is expected or unexpected.*

Assessment Finding	Expected	Not Expected
1:1 A-P transverse diameter		
Oxygenation saturation 93%		
Respiratory rate 28		
Rhonchi upon auscultation		

Answer/Rationale:

Assessment Finding	Expected	Not Expected
1:1 A-P transverse diameter	X	
Oxygenation saturation 93%	X	
Respiratory rate 28		X
Rhonchi upon auscultation		X

An A-P transverse ratio of 1:1 indicate barrel chest. While this is not a normal finding, it is anticipated in patients with longstanding chronic bronchitis as pulmonary remodeling takes place. In a patient with no disease, a 1:2 ratio is expected. An oxygen saturation of 93% is an expected finding in chronic bronchitis, as patients live in a hypoxic, hypercapnic state. In patients with no history of respiratory disease, an O2 saturation of > 95% should be expected. A respiratory rate of 28 is elevated and may indicate an exacerbation of chronic bronchitis. Rhonchi indicate increased mucous in the airways and might also be a sign of exacerbation.

6. Hot spot

A 22-year-old patient presents to the urgent care clinic with complaints of fever and abdominal pain. She is concerned she might have appendicitis. Pain felt in which area of the abdomen most strongly suggests inflammation of the appendix? *Place an 'x' in the correct region.*

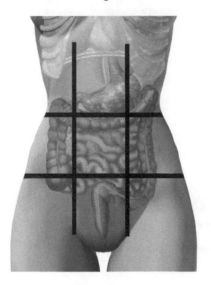

Answer/Rationale:

The appendix is located in the right iliac region of the abdomen. Pain related to inflammation of the appendix is most often felt in this area.

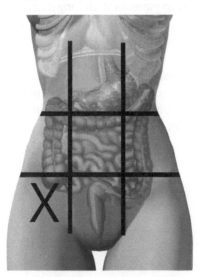

7. Cloze

A patient whose LMP was on July 17th, 2023, presents for complaints of abdominal fullness. During her exam, the cervix is noted to have a bluish color consistent with ___1___ . Additionally, the cervix has softened, indicating a positive ___2___ . A positive urine ___3___ determines the patient is pregnant. The nurse calculates the estimated date of delivery to be ___4___ .

Complete the sentence using the following options.

1. Chadwick's sign, Goodell's sign, Hegar's sign
2. Chadwick's sign, Goodell's sign, Hegar's sign
3. HCG, protein, ketone
4. April 24th, 2024; March 3rd, 2024; February 3rd, 2024

Answer/Rationale:
1. **Chadwick's sign:** The bluish discoloration of the cervix that develops after six to eight weeks of pregnancy.
2. **Goodell's sign:** The softening of the cervix as a consequence of increased hormone production.
3. **HCG:** Human chorionic gonadotropin is a hormone detectable in blood and urine that rises with pregnancy.
4. **April 24th, 2024:** Nagel's rule is used to calculate the estimated date of delivery.

   July – 3 months = April

   17 + 7 days = 24

   Next year 2024

8. Extended multiple response

The nurse is evaluating a new skin lesion. Which qualities of the lesion increase the nurse's suspicion of malignancy? *(Select all that apply)*

A) Irregular borders
B) Diameter 9 mm
C) Brown coloration
D) Ragged borders
E) Lesion symmetry
F) Stable appearance since last visit

Answer: A, B, D

9. Matrix

A patient is diagnosed with a thyroid goiter. They are undergoing further evaluation for possible thyroid dysfunction. Which signs and symptoms should the nurse associate with hypothyroidism or hyperthyroidism? *Place an 'x' in the matrix to indicate if the sign/symptom is found in hypothyroidism or hyperthyroidism.*

Sign/Symptom	Hypothyroidism	Hyperthyroidism
Weight gain		
Cold intolerance		
Heart palpitations		
Dry skin		
Tremor		

Answer:

Sign/Symptom	Hypothyroidism	Hyperthyroidism
Weight gain	X	
Cold intolerance	X	
Heart palpitations		X
Dry skin	X	
Tremor		X

10. Extended multiple response

The nurse caring for a transgender patient notes bruising on the patient's wrists and back. Which assessment does the nurse prioritize for this patient?

A) Screen for IPV

B) Assess the blood pressure

C) Administer a PHQ-9 questionnaire

D) Inspect for equal chest expansion

E) Palpate the point of maximal impulse (PMI)

Answer: A

Index

K

kidney infections, 202–205

Korotkoff sounds, 52

L

language, fluency, 47

layers of skin, 216

learning

    active, 2

    comparing to understanding, 1

lentigo senilis (liver spots), 220, 220*f*

lesbians, 254, 256

lesions, 217

LGBTQIA+ community, 260. *See also* transgender patients

lice, 222

lifts, 145

listening, active, 71

literature, evidence-based, 3

lithotomy position, 209, 210*f*

liver

    function of, 187–188

    gastroenterological anomalies, 182–183

    risk factors for disease, 180

liver spots (lentigo senilis), 220, 220*f*

living children, number of, 205

locations

    of murmurs, 143

    of pulse, 147*f*

logic, 84–85

long-term (remote) memory, 82

low-fidelity simulations, 3

lungs. *See also* respiratory anomalies

    anterior-posterior (A-P) diameter, 165–168

    right middle lobe of, 161

    view of, 160*f*, 161*f*

M

macules, 228*t*

Mankoski Pain Scale, 177*t*

Maslow's hierarchy of needs, 35–38, 36*f*

measurements. *See also* vital sign assessment

    blood pressure, 51–52 (*see also* blood pressure)

    NCJMM (NCSBN Clinical Judgment Measurement Model), 22

    pupillary dilation, 124*f*

medical histories, 104

Medical Research Council Manual Muscle Testing Scale, 129–130

medication reconciliations, 96

melanin, 216

melanoma, 218, 220–222

melena, 185–186, 185*t*

memory, 82–84, 89–99. *See also* geriatric patients

mental status assessment, 71

    behaviors, 73–76

    cognition, 82–86

    insight, 86–88

    Mini-Mental Status Examination (MMSE), 132, 133*f*

    observation, 71–73

    perceptions, 80–82

    responses to cognitive questions, 85–86

    thought content, 78–80

    thought process, 76–78

metoidioplasty, 253

Mini-Mental Status Examination (MMSE), 132, 133*f*

miosis, causes of, 125

miotic pupillary responses, 125*f*

mistakes in interviews, 44–45

mnemonics, 196–197, 229

models, NCJMM (NCSBN Clinical Judgment Measurement Model), 22

modifiable risk factors, 120

moles, presence of, 218

mood, 73, 74*t*

multiple choice questions, 16

multiple response questions, 16–17

murmurs, 142, 145

    classifying graded, 143*t*

    intensity, 143